Intermittent Fasting for Women Over 50

A Guide to Feeling Healthier, Younger, and More Energetic

Gabriel Baker

Contents

A Special Gift to Our Readers

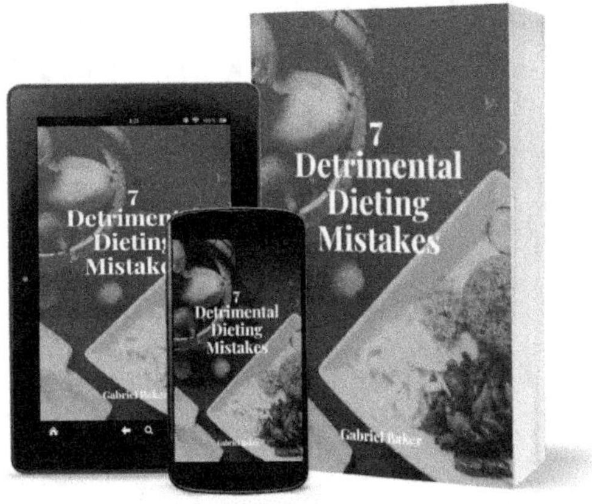

Included with your purchase of this book is our 7 Detrimental Dieting Mistakes List. This list will run through some of the most common and grave dieting mistakes and help you in maintaining a successful diet by giving you solutions to your dieting problems.

Click the link below and let us know which email to deliver it to.

gabriel-baker.com

Introduction

Together with a host of symptoms that usher in menopause, women in their 50s have to contend with weight gain, mostly around the midsection, a slowed-down metabolism, and mood swings. Even though this happens mainly due to a hormonal imbalance that takes place at this stage of life, there are other factors at play, such as one's lifestyle, aging, and genetic factors. Weight gain around the midsection is a great cause for concern because it increases your risk of other health conditions such as type 2 diabetes, breathing problems, and heart and blood vessel diseases. During this phase of life, you may also be at risk of certain cancers, like breast, colon, and endometrial.

Did you know that obesity and overweight contributed to 4 million deaths in 2017? The World Health Organization (WHO) estimates that the problem of obesity and overweight affects 42% of the U.S. population. This increases slightly to 44% in the 40–59-year age group (CDC, 2022). What is shocking about these statistics is that things don't have to be this way. This is a totally preventable problem. The point of sharing these statistics is not to scare you as a woman in this age bracket but to shed some light on the issue and offer some solutions. One of those solutions is adjusting your lifestyle, and by lifestyle, we are talking specifically about your diet, which you have total control over. Exercise is also another solution that we are all familiar with, but not everyone is able to exercise for various reasons which are beyond the scope of this book.

So the objective of this book is two-pronged: firstly, to introduce intermittent fasting (IF) as a potential solution by sharing as much information as possible about it, not only as a weight loss tool but as a lifestyle that offers you many other health benefits that a woman in her 50s and beyond would only be too happy to learn about, and secondly, to give you practical tools that you can start using today to get you started on your IF journey.

Some topics we will cover throughout this book are the following:

- *What IF is and its health benefits*. There is a lot of misinformation about what IF is, and in this book, I will present some facts and even back them up with a bit of science, so you can be assured that I am not making things up.
- *What IF does or doesn't do for women*. In case you are wondering if women gain the same benefits as men on IF, Chapter 2 will answer that question.
- *IF after 50*. You may be wondering, *At my age, is it not too late to start IF? What could be the benefits?* Chapter 4 will answer those specific questions.
- *The different IF plans*. Too many choices can be confusing; let's help you decide what's good for you.
- *What foods to eat while IF*. I've got you covered. I provide a long list of foods to choose from, so you can never run out of choices.
- *How to get started*. Here, I share some practical tools to prepare you mentally and physically to start IF.

- *The interplay between IF and exercise.* To exercise or not to exercise? What does science say?
- *Meal planning.* I share a few examples of meal plans here to guide you in designing your own.
- *IF recipes.* In Chapter 9, I share lots of recipes that I know you will love. Remember, these can be tweaked to your preference too.
- *Debunking some myths around IF.* What are some of the myths you have heard about IF? Let's talk about them, and hopefully, I can help put your mind at ease.

At this point, you are probably wondering who I am and what makes me an authority on this subject. When I was 6 years old, my family moved from the Netherlands to the UK, and I have been living there since. I was diagnosed with gut issues and had to change my diet to overcome that. I have since become very passionate about sharing this knowledge and experience to help others struggling with the same condition. I realize that many people suffer from chronic diseases and want an easy-to-follow guide to help them adopt a new diet, overcome their disease, and live a healthy lifestyle. Because I have always been an inquisitive person, wanting to learn and implement what I have learned to help others, I decided to write this book. I hope that this book will help you overcome the barriers to changing your diet and help you take that first step to a healthier lifestyle, free from diseases and constant medication.

Next Steps

Admitting that there is a problem is the first step, and I'm guessing that you picked this book up because you realize that you could use some help. However, admitting on its own doesn't fix the problem. The next step is the most crucial step, and that is information gathering. So to help you with that next step, in the following chapter, we will go into great detail about what IF is and isn't. Hopefully, this will help you sift out the misinformation you may have picked up from the *not-so-reliable* sources about IF and help you decide if it's the best tool to achieve your health goals. Finally, I wish to close this chapter with this famous quote:

You are only one defining decision away from a totally different life!

— Mark Batterson

I know you can't wait to get started, so let's hop on to Chapter 1.

Chapter 1: What Is Intermittent Fasting?

Intermittent fasting (IF) is a way of eating where a person cycles between periods of eating and fasting. Throughout this book, you will hear me referring to them as *eating windows* and *fasting windows*. IF has its roots in traditional fasting that is practiced in some cultures for religious or spiritual reasons. This way of eating has become very popular in the healthy lifestyle community in recent years. One of the best things about IF is that it comes with a variety of plans to choose from, so when a person decides to embark on the IF journey, they would choose a schedule or plan most suitable to their lifestyle. We will go into detail about the individual plans in Chapter 3. There are many health benefits that IF presents, one of them being that when you fast, your body regulates its hormone production, making the stored fat more accessible to be burned off. We will discuss the mechanics of this a bit later on. The other health benefit is that during the fasting period, your cells initiate important repair processes and change the expression of genes in the body. Again, more on this to follow.

Prolonged fasting prompts our bodies to initiate a process called *ketosis*. Ketosis is referred to by scientists as the "metabolic switching" state, and this is when the body starts breaking down fat for fuel, using stored fatty acids instead of glycogen for energy. Let me break this down a bit more: Normally, when we eat, our bodies store glucose as glycogen to supply it with energy throughout the day. When we burn through the glycogen stores until they are depleted, as a result of fasting, the body looks for the next source of energy, and that is when it switches to burning the stored fat. Cue in *ketosis*.

The above are just a few examples of how IF benefits your health. We will discuss these in detail in the next sections.

What Are the Advantages of IF?

IF Supports Weight Loss

When we restrict the number of hours we consume food during the day, this directly restricts our calorie intake. However, this can only happen if you eat *normally* during the eating window, and by this, I mean not overeating to make up for the hours you were fasting. Overeating during the eating window will negate the effects of fasting. Scientific studies have shown that IF can trigger a weight loss of anything between 2.5% and 9.9% of body weight (Stockman et al., 2018).

The other mechanism through which IF helps you lose weight is by increasing your metabolism. It has been demonstrated, through research, that IF increases metabolism, in some cases, by up to 14% (Netshiomvani, 2022). When your metabolism is increased, the body burns fat faster.

Thirdly, when you eat, your body produces a hormone called insulin. Insulin's main function is to regulate glucose (blood sugar) in your body, and it does this by breaking it down and transporting it to the cells, where it will be stored as glycogen for later use. Decreasing the number of times you eat during the day decreases the number of times insulin is produced by the body, which directly translates to less glycogen stored up. Glycogen is a carbohydrate; it is the stored form of glucose that supplies the body with energy, as briefly discussed in the section above. When glycogen is present in the body, the body cannot burn fat until it has burned through its glycogen stores. Fasting helps you to burn through these glycogen stores faster, and when this happens, the body looks for the next source of energy which is fat. That's when it can start burning through the stored fat. And this is how you lose weight.

Reversal of Type 2 Diabetes

I'm going to talk about the role of insulin, here again, so bear with me. The pancreas produces insulin in the body. In the above section, we already mentioned that the role of insulin is to transport glucose into the cells, and that's how it maintains a normal blood sugar level in a person's body. You have probably heard the term *insulin resistance* and may or may not know what it means. Simply put, with some people, when insulin transports glucose into the cells, the cells resist this process, not allowing glucose to enter, which then causes a buildup of insulin in the bloodstream. This triggers the pancreas to produce more insulin, and it does this until it can't produce anymore. At this point, you would be diagnosed as *insulin resistant*. IF reverses this process because it regulates how much insulin is produced by the pancreas, and this allows the body enough time to burn through its glucose stores to get to the fat stores. A lot of research has been done in this area including a study done in men with prediabetes who showed significant improvements in insulin sensitivity after being put through an IF regime (Sutton et al., 2018). A study done in women showed a 19% decrease in insulin resistance and 29% lower insulin levels over a period of six months on IF (Harvie et al., 2010).

IF Lowers the Bad Cholesterol

There is evidence that IF lowers the bad cholesterol in the body. A systematic review of studies looking at the relationship between IF and its effects on cholesterol showed significant improvements in total cholesterol as well as low-density lipoprotein (LDL), which is the bad cholesterol (Meng et al., 2020).

Similar results were found in an earlier review that was done in 2018 (Santos & Macedo, 2018).

IF Increases Growth Hormone

IF has been shown to improve the production of human growth hormone (HGH). Some studies have shown that HGH can be improved by up to 300% after three days of fasting (Ho et al., 1988). HGH is responsible for enhancing collagen production that is responsible for healthy nails, hair, and joints. HGH plays a role in stimulating fat burning, improving muscle development and bone density, reducing inflammation, and improving immune coordination (Jockers, 2019).

IF Reduces Inflammation

Inflammation was significantly reduced in a group of study participants who were fasting during Ramadan (Faris et al., 2012). These findings were only observed during the fasting period compared to when the subjects were not fasting. One obvious way in which fasting helps to reduce inflammation is through hydration. Fasting causes one to increase their water intake, and as hydration increases, this helps to fight off free radicals in the body, ultimately leading to less inflammation. Free radicals cause aging and other illnesses in the body.

More recently, research done by Malinowski et al. (2019) showed that IF also reduced concentrations of pro-inflammatory markers such as homocysteine, interleukin-6 (IL-6), and C-reactive protein

(CRP). These cause prolonged inflammation which potentially leads to diseases such as atherosclerosis, heart disease, osteoporosis, and diabetes (Hanka, 2021).

IF Promotes Heart Health

IF improves cardiovascular (heart) health. A recent study showed that IF "lowered resting heart rate and reduced systolic and diastolic arterial blood pressures, as well as pulse pressure and pulse wave velocity" (Stekovic et al., 2019). An earlier study done by Varady et al. (2009) showed that IF was effective in reducing coronary artery disease (CAD) in adults with obesity who were put on a 10-week trial, eight weeks of which was on IF. IF does this by lowering blood pressure, triglycerides, and LDL, which are all drivers of poor heart health. These results were confirmed in another study by Mattson et al. (2017).

IF Prevents Aging

Here, I want to talk briefly about a process called *autophagy*. From the Greek *auto,* which means "self", and *phagy,* which means "cleaning," the word *autophagy* means "self-cleaning." This is a process by which the body cleans itself, a process that, according to some scientists, takes place 24 hours after calorie restriction has been initiated (Jamshed et al., 2019). During fasting, this can only happen once the glycogen stores are extremely low in the body. When the body reaches this state, it begins to create new cells, and it gets rid of old or dysfunctional ones, which, when you think about it, is the antiaging effect of IF. So what autophagy does is help the body repair itself. Similarly, studies have shown that autophagy helps fight off neurodegenerative diseases such as Parkinson's and Alzheimer's, and it does this by removing toxic proteins from within the cells that contribute to neurodegenerative diseases (Glick et al., 2010).

The other way in which fasting contributes to antiaging is through the production of a ketone called *beta-hydroxybutyrate.* This ketone is produced during ketosis, and its main function is to trigger the multiplication of youthful cells in the body. In lab rats, fasting was shown to improve their life span by up to 83% compared to other diets, more confirmation of its antiaging effects of IF (Mattson et al., 2017).

IF Improves Brain Health

Fasting can enhance cognitive function. This was shown in earlier studies on mice (Li et al., 2013) and later confirmed in human studies (Anton et al., 2018). It does this by triggering the production of a hormone called *brain-derived neurotrophic factor* (BDNF). This hormone improves concentration and mental flexibility. Low amounts of BDNF are linked to poor brain health and, in some cases, depression.

We have already mentioned above how IF, through the process of autophagy, helps fight off neurodegenerative diseases like epilepsy, Parkinson's, and Alzheimer's because of its *cleaning* properties, again, more confirmation of its positive effects on brain health.

IF Improves Gut Health

There are three ways in which IF does this. The first is through hydration. As you increase your water intake, it helps the body to flush out toxic cells and the bacteria, which greatly improves your gut health.

The second way that IF improves your gut health is through the improvement of the microbiome (the presence of certain microorganisms) in the gut. Both good and bad bacteria exist in your gut, but removing food assists in increasing a certain specific bacteria known as *Akkermansia muciniphila*. This is the bacteria that contributes to lowering inflammation in the body, which directly improves your gut health.

Thirdly, IF works with your circadian rhythm, or your body clock, to improve gut health. Scientific studies show that bacteria also have their own circadian rhythm, and this suggests that some bacteria are more active at night while some function during the day, so eating at night messes up the functioning of these bacteria.

IF Improves Confidence

A group of 52 women with a mean age of 25 reported that IF improved their sense of achievement, reward, pride, and control over their lives, even though they reported being significantly hungrier and more irritable at the end of their fasting (Watkins & Serpell, 2016). This is a clear indication of the positive psychological effects of IF.

The Disadvantages of IF

You're Likely to Feel Hungry on IF

When you are someone who is used to eating three or more meals a day, which most people are, you may struggle with maintaining fasting periods. The good news is that even though it may be challenging in the initial stages, you do eventually get used to going for certain periods without eating. You will develop your *fasting muscle*. This may require a certain level of discipline on your part or finding other means to deal with your hunger pangs, which we will talk about a bit later on in the book. The important thing is to remember that it is normal to feel hungry in the beginning. Increased hunger pangs during fasting were also reported in a year-long study that compared IF with other calorie-restricted regimens (Sundfør et al., 2018). So, you are not alone. Take heart.

Practicing IF Is Likely to Go Against Your Intuition

In relation to the above, if you are used to eating at certain specific times, your body prompts you that it is now time to eat, so it may feel like you are going against your intuition that tells you when it's time to eat. Following a schedule could also be frustrating to people who are intuitive eaters, but as we have already mentioned, this will come with a bit of practice and self-discipline.

You May Experience Headaches Especially in the Initial Stages

This is likely to be the case at the beginning, as your body starts experiencing lower blood sugar levels and you are adjusting to a new eating schedule. There are ways to deal with and overcome this. Most people report minor problems like headaches, nausea, and bloating in the first three days of starting IF, and these eventually go away. Please allow yourself to eat something small if you are really struggling; however, if the headaches won't go away, please consult a health practitioner for a checkup and/or advice.

Some people also report irritability (Watkins & Serpell, 2016) and feeling a bit *out of sorts*. It is important to remember that these are just *teething problems* that will go away if you persevere.

IF Could Lead to Weight Gain

Some people complain that IF causes them to gain weight, but often, this is because they are making the simple mistake of binging during the eating periods. We briefly mentioned this at the beginning of the chapter that if you overeat, you will negate the effects of IF because by doing so, you will be increasing your calorie intake. When you increase your calorie intake, you are more likely to go over your daily limit. Remember, the formula to lose weight is to *burn more calories than what you are taking in*.

Another culprit that has been found to cause weight gain in those who practice IF is too much caffeine. Research shows that too much caffeine can lead to weight gain by increasing blood glucose levels. In this study, consuming too much caffeine decreased insulin sensitivity in some people by up to 37% (Whitehead & White, 2013).

To reiterate what was said earlier in the chapter, less insulin sensitivity means less likely to burn fat.

You May Experience Nutrient Deficiencies

Eating the *wrong* foods during your eating window will lead to nutrient deficiencies in the body. Some people take the *eat anything you like* during eating periods too much to heart and assume that they can eat a whole pizza and wash it down with a bottle of wine. If you do that, your body will not get the nutrients that it requires to meet all of its bodily functions. Your body is supposed to be getting the required and daily recommended amounts of protein, carbs, and vitamins, including other micronutrients. This can only be achieved by eating wholesome foods that meet those needs.

IF Could Reduce Physical Activity

There are some concerns that IF could lead to reduced physical activity. This concern is based on the assumption that you will not have enough energy to exercise while you are fasting. There are studies that have also shown that IF may impair exercise performance (Kerksick et al., 2017) and lead to light-headedness because of lowered blood pressure and blood sugar levels. Research in this area has come up with conflicting information as some have shown great benefits of combining exercise with IF, including increased energy levels. Some have shown that combining IF with exercise leads to even more weight loss (Bhutani et al., 2013) and triggers autophagy (Jaspers et al., 2016). This is great news for those who love to exercise.

IF Can Lead to the Development of Eating Disorders

Any type of restrictive eating or calorie reduction has the potential to trigger eating disorders, especially in those who are susceptible to acquiring those disorders. It is always advisable to seek the opinion of a health practitioner before getting started on any diet because they would be in a better position to advise you based on your medical history.

Since IF *trains* you to go for long periods without food, some people might start pushing themselves to extremes to see how long they can go without, and this is dangerous for one's health as the body will suffer from nutritional deficiency.

IF Is Not Suitable for Those Who Are on Medications

Those who are on medications usually have to take them at certain specified times, and most meds have to be taken with food. IF does not work well with this, as one cannot take medicines while fasting. If you are on chronic medication, it is advisable that you speak to your healthcare provider before starting IF.

In this chapter, we have discussed the many benefits or advantages of adopting IF as a lifestyle, and hopefully, by now, you will realize that there is a lot to be gained from it. We have, however, also noted that there are some disadvantages, albeit fewer, but still caution should be exercised. I also want to emphasize the importance of speaking to your healthcare practitioner if you are not sure if you are the right candidate for IF.

In the next chapter, we drill down to what benefits IF has for women specifically.

Chapter 2: Intermittent Fasting for Women

Firstly, we know that almost all diets affect men and women differently. IF is the same, and this is why this book is geared toward women specifically. Some differences that have been observed between men and women who practice IF are around bone health, reproductive health, and overall well-being.

In this chapter, we are going to go into detail about how IF affects women compared to men. According to ISSA (2022), "gender roles dictated by biology have played a part in shaping male and female metabolic responses to exercise, carbohydrates, sleep deprivation, and yes—you guessed it—fasting." They claim that the way men's and women's bodies respond to fasting dates back to how their bodies were adapted for the hunter-gatherer times, where men's bodies responded with a boost in metabolic rate during fasting and women's responded with a decreased metabolism as the body slowed down to conserve energy. This is still evident in today's society and can be observed during IF.

At this point, I also wish to caution that if you are someone who is already living with diabetes or taking some kind of medication, it will be very important that you seek the medical opinion of your doctor to assess if you would be a good candidate for IF before you embark on this journey.

The Benefits of IF for Women

Weight Loss

Studies show that IF is an effective method for weight loss in older women. One particular study showed a significant weight loss of around 4.5 lb (2 kg) in women over 60 years of age after they followed the 16:8 plan (more on the plans later) for six weeks (Domaszewski et al., 2020).

In a lab study that compared male and female rats on five different eating plans, including IF, the females who were put on the IF and 20% calorie-restricted diets showed similar body weight responses to males than on the three other plans. Females also consumed less food than their counterparts across all five feeding protocols (Martin et al., 2007).

In a different study, looking at weight loss specifically, IF significantly decreased belly fat, in some cases, by as much as 7% (Barnosky et al., 2014a). Why is this important for you? Research shows that belly fat may pose more danger for women than it does for men (Harvard Health Publishing, 2021a). In a study that followed half a million people aged 40–69 over a period of seven years, the women who carried more weight around their middle had a 10%–20% higher risk of heart attack than those who didn't at baseline. These researchers concluded that a waist-to-hip ratio was 18% stronger as a predictor of heart attacks in women than in men, where it was 6% by comparison.

Are you curious to know what your waist-to-hip ratio is? It is a very simple calculation that you do by dividing your waist measurement by your hip measurement. A healthy waist-to-hip measurement for women should not exceed 0.86, and for men, this should be 1.00.

What Is the Role of Hormones?

IF May Affect Your Reproductive Health

I know that this may not be a concern for a woman in her 50s and above, but it's still worth a mention, especially if you are a woman who's raising girls. It is important to note that most of the studies that have been done looking specifically at reproductive health have been done in female rodents, where the results showed that IF may cause changes in estrogen levels. This obviously has a direct negative impact on reproductive functions such as the menstrual cycle, fertility, pregnancy, and lactation (Martin et al., 2009).

So what this means is that IF might cause you to miss your periods, again, that is if you are someone who is still getting her menses. This, according to Dr. Woitowich (Jarreau, 2020), is because "extreme forms of caloric restriction, weight loss, exercise, and nutritional deficiencies can all cause amenorrhea, or irregular or skipped periods." Caloric restriction impacts the production of sex hormones through the hypothalamic–pituitary–gonadal (HPG) axis, which then leads to irregular menses. So those who are planning to become pregnant in the future should exercise caution because the body starts preparing for pregnancy right at the beginning of puberty, and this lasts throughout a woman's reproductive years.

What About the Role of Hormones Outside of Reproductive Health?

Studies done in women have shown an increase in cortisol, the stress hormone, and less insulin sensitivity during IF (ISSA, 2022). We should remember that since cortisol is the stress hormone, it will be important to maintain a healthy lifestyle to fight off stress. In people who were placed on a 48-hour fast, the results showed that "men became more parasympathetic from fasting, meaning their nervous system was less agitated, whereas women became more sympathetic, meaning their bodies were more stressed, more in the 'fight or flight' state" (Solianik et al., 2016; Solianik & Sujeta, 2018).

We also know that IF lowers ghrelin, the hormone that signals the body when it is hungry. Leptin and ghrelin are the two hunger hormones, but the two act in opposition to one another. Ghrelin's function is to signal hunger or stimulate appetite, and leptin regulates appetite by telling the body when it is full, so you can stop eating. It turns out that women have higher levels of leptin compared with men (Dornbush & Aeddula, 2020). This is really good news because it indicates that women reach levels of satiety much faster than men.

Glucose Levels and Insulin in the Blood

A study that compared men's and women's blood glucose levels after a 38-hour fast showed the blood glucose levels of women to be significantly lower compared to those of men (Soeters et al., 2007). Another study that followed a group of premenopausal women overweight and obess for a period of six months compared IF to a calorie-restricted diet and found that even though both protocols reduced fasting insulin and insulin resistance, IF did a better job than the other diet. In this study, insulin levels were reduced by 29% and insulin resistance by 19% (Harvie et al., 2010).

Another study that enrolled both men and women on an alternate-day fasting (ADF) regimen showed differences between the genders in their glucose responses and insulin levels. In women, the glucose response was slightly impaired, and the insulin remained unchanged after 22 days, but there was no change in glucose in men, even though a significant reduction in insulin was observed (Heilbronn, Civitarese, et al., 2005). The scientists concluded that these results meant that IF might affect glucose tolerance in women but not in men. Despite the not-so-stellar performance of IF in this study, a reduction in insulin is still great news when it comes to reducing the risk of diabetes.

Even though the data seems to be a bit mixed in terms of whether IF affects insulin differently for men versus women, one thing that we see consistently is that IF has a positive impact on insulin and blood sugar management. The research is mixed because most of these studies are small, and most of them do not go to the lengths of teasing out gender differences. You are therefore advised to exercise caution with regard to how you interpret these results.

Autophagy

In lab rats, males experienced more autophagy than female rats, but this has not been confirmed in human studies yet.

Cancer

IF may prevent the development of certain cancers in women. Cancer is one of the leading causes of morbidity and mortality in the world, and in women, breast cancer, for instance, is the second most common cancer in the world. In a review of different studies, the researchers concluded that fasting has protective benefits against certain cancers because of how it decreases the biomarkers or risk factors for cancer (Nair & Khawale, 2016). One of the studies cited in that report showed that IF inhibits tumor growth by inhibiting angiogenesis. Angiogenesis is the growth of new blood vessels that leads to tumor growth.

Cardiovascular Health

The WHO reports that around 17.9 million deaths occur yearly as a result of cardiovascular diseases and that these mostly affect people above the age of 45 (World Health Organization, 2021b). Even though more men than women die in the 45–59 age group, women's deaths surpass men's in the 60 and above age group. Sadly, these are mainly caused by a certain lifestyle and so, by their nature, are preventable diseases. Scientists say that gender differences are related to the cardioprotective effects of estrogen in premenopausal women. In a systematic review of the literature, the scientists concluded that IF limits many risk factors that lead to the development of cardiovascular diseases (CVDs). They also concluded that IF decreases the risk for atherosclerosis, the buildup of plaque in the walls of the arteries. It does this by reducing the concentration of inflammatory markers, such as IL-6, homocysteine, and CRP (Malinowski et al., 2019).

Cholesterol

Still under the subject of heart health, cholesterol is one of the leading risk factors for heart health. Women seem to do better when it comes to cholesterol regulation than men on IF. Significant improvements in HDL were observed among women participants in a study that compared men's and women's lipid profiles after IF (Santos & Macedo, 2018), so this is definitely good news for women. Similar results were shown in another study that enrolled 12 women and 4 men who had obesity. In this study, both total cholesterol and LDL decreased while HDL remained unchanged, a demonstration that IF delivers great benefits when it comes to cholesterol regulation (Varady et al., 2009). This is further confirmation that women do better on heart health matters than men do when they practice IF.

High Blood Pressure

Another big risk factor for cardiovascular health is hypertension, also known as high blood pressure. Hypertension affects nearly half of all adults living in the US (CDC, 2020b). This is something that places them at huge risk for heart disease and stroke, both leading causes of death in the US. The CDC reports that only a quarter of those living with this condition have it under control. Even though it affects men more than women and certain racial groups than others, you may still be at risk and therefore wondering if there's anything that IF can do for you. Well, I have good news for you. In a study done by Baylor College of Medicine in which they looked at the effect of IF in the gut, they showed that fasting lowers blood pressure by reshaping the composition of the gut microbiota (microorganisms that are found in the gut) (Shi et al., 2021).

Bone Health

There is some research that suggests that IF may negatively impact bone strength and bone density, but these are studies that were carried out in rodents (Hisatomi & Kugino, 2019). A review of studies that compared IF to other calorie-restricted diets showed that IF did not impact bone mineral density as much as the other diets did (Veronese & Reginster, 2019). These are small studies, and the results should be interpreted with great caution. This means that larger studies are required to confirm this.

What Types of Women Should Not Try IF?

Women who fall under the following categories should not practice IF:

- planning to fall pregnant or lactating women
- those who are living with diabetes (unless they confirm with their doctor first)
- those who have fertility problems
- those who are underweight, malnourished, or have nutritional deficiencies
- those who have a history of eating disorders

IF has a good safety profile, but if you experience alarming symptoms such as loss of menstrual cycle, you should definitely stop doing it and seek the advice of a doctor.

To sum up the discussion above, I want to end this chapter by noting the many health benefits that IF has for women, which makes it a great tool for weight loss and health in general, as this section has demonstrated. I also want to caution here that although there are gender differences noted in some studies, please exercise caution in how you interpret these results as most of the research that has been done in humans has enrolled mostly male participants, and so we should be careful about generalizing the results to the female population.

Chapter 3: The Different Types of Intermittent Fasting

In the previous chapters, you've heard me referring to IF plans or methods, and in this chapter, we are going to discuss the various plans that I promised to go into detail about later. We are also going to talk about the best ones for women. Once you have this information, you will be in a better position to choose the one that is best for you.

The Different Types of IF

The first thing you need to know is that there are three main categories that IF plans or schedules fall into, and these are alternate-day fasting (ADF), periodic fasting, and time-restricted feeding (TRF), also known as early time-restricted feeding (eTRF).

Alternate-Day Fasting

As the name suggests, ADF is the plan where you fast every alternative day, so you would eat normally every other day. Most people seem to agree that this is the easiest plan to do. The ADF can also be modified for those who cannot go on a full day without eating. In the modified version, you are allowed to eat a maximum of 500 calories on your fasting days, if you are a woman (for men, this is 600). On your non-fasting days, please make sure that you do not overeat to make up for the fasting days. We already discussed the negative effects of doing this in the previous chapters.

The Benefits of ADF

The ADF method has been studied extensively, and it was proven to be very effective in inducing weight loss in adults with obesity (Catenacci et al., 2016), improving heart health, reducing fat mass (particularly the trunk fat), improving the fat-to-lean ratio, and fighting the aging process (Stekovic et al., 2019). Combining ADF with strength training can help you lose twice as much weight as doing ADF on its own and six times as much weight loss as doing exercise alone (Bhutani et al., 2013). We will discuss the role of exercise in detail in Chapter 7.

Another study showed that ADF increased the levels of brain-derived neurotrophic factor (BDNF) when compared to other calorie-restriction diets (Catenacci et al., 2016). We mentioned BDNF in the previous chapter under brain health as the hormone that improves concentration and mental flexibility.

Those who have been on ADF report that this method does not increase *compensatory hunger*, the increased hunger that is a direct response to calorie restrictions. So if you are concerned that you will experience increased hunger while on this plan, this is not the case. In fact, most people report that their hunger diminishes after the initial two weeks of being on ADF.

One of the main benefits of the ADF method is that it has been shown to reverse many symptoms of type 2 diabetes in people who are overweight and obese (Barnosky et al., 2014b). ADF also works for people within a *normal* weight range as this one study showed that over a three-week period, people experienced increased fat burn, decreased insulin, and showed a 4% decrease in fat mass (Heilbronn, Smith, et al., 2005). Because the ADF method provides less calories than what one actually needs to maintain weight, it may not be suitable for those who are not looking to lose fat mass.

One of the concerns that have been raised about the ADF plan is that it may induce *starvation mode* in the body. Starvation mode is when the body responds to calorie restriction by slowing down its metabolic rate to conserve energy. When this happens, the body reduces the number of calories that it burns. Research has shown that this is not the case with ADF. A study that compared the ADF method to other calorie-restricted diets showed that while these diets significantly decreased the metabolic rate by 6%, the ADF method only reduced it by an insignificant 1% (Catenacci et al., 2016).

So What to Eat on the ADF?

The main thing to remember here is what we mentioned earlier, to not take the *eat whatever you like* advice too literally so as not to sabotage your weight loss efforts. If you are on the *modified ADF*, you have to ensure that you stay within the 500-calorie limit on your fasting days. I have recipes to help you with this in Chapter 9. Also, make sure that you can stay hydrated by drinking as much as you like of the zero-calorie drinks; think tea, black coffee, and water. With food specifically, always choose highly nutritious foods like chicken, eggs, fish, high-quality dairy, etc. These provide your body with high-quality proteins. Do not forget to also load up on low- or zero-calorie vegetables such as the dark leafy types and tomatoes. Remember, you can also make soups with your vegetables, especially on cold days when you don't feel like eating a salad.

Is ADF Safe?

The ADF plan has been tested in different studies and found to be safe for most people. It also does not cause weight regain when compared to other calorie-restricted diets. It is important to note that the ADF method has not been tested on pregnant women and those with a history of eating disorders, and so it is not advisable for those groups of people to go on it without consulting their health practitioner. ADF is also not recommended for the following populations: lactating women, children younger than 18 years, those who are underweight, and those with medical conditions.

Lastly, my advice to those who would like to try this plan out is to test both the modified and the unmodified versions at the beginning to see which one suits you better. That way, you will have more chances of being successful on this plan.

Periodic Fasting

The 5:2 Method

Made popular by Dr. Michael Mosley, a British journalist, this method was first introduced by Dr. Jason Fung, author of the book *The Obesity Code*. The 5:2 method is also called *The Fast Diet*. In this method, you eat for five days and fast for two nonconsecutive days of the week. So before you start on it, you should decide which days you will fast and which days you will eat normally. With this method too, you are allowed to eat 500 calories a day on your fasting days on the modified plan. This might be the simplest diet protocol to observe, and many people report that they find it easier to stick to.

The Benefits of the 5:2 Method

Few studies have been done on the 5:2 method specifically, although it is expected that it carries the same benefits as other IF methods. A study that followed premenopausal women who were overweight or obese over a period of six months showed that the 5:2 method was just as effective at inducing weight loss as other calorie-restrictive diets and in improving insulin sensitivity. The two groups also showed comparable reductions in leptin, total and LDL cholesterol, as well as blood pressure (Harvie et al., 2010).

The alternative to the 5:2 method is the 4:3 method. This method has been shown to reduce insulin resistance, asthma, allergies, heart arrhythmias, and even menopausal hot flashes (Johnson et al., 2006; Bjarnadottir, 2018). In a randomized controlled trial (RCT), the 4:3 plan demonstrated great success at reducing body weight by up to 11 lb, fat mass by 7.7 lb, triglycerides by 20%, and leptin levels by 40% (Varady et al., 2013).

A modified version of the 5:2 method tested in a group of people overweight and obese showed that it was just as effective as other calorie-restrictive methods in reducing visceral fat mass, fasting insulin, and insulin resistance. The scientists behind this study concluded that the IF method showed promise as an alternative diet method for weight loss and for type 2 diabetes risk reduction in those overweight and obese (Barnosky et al., 2014a).

So What to Eat on the 5:2?

On this plan, you can choose whether you prefer to schedule your meals a little earlier in the day; as an example, you could have a small breakfast and a larger meal a little later in the day, or you could have your first meal of the day a bit later, and this could be anywhere between 10 a.m. and noon and then your next meal in the late afternoon or early evening. Some people opt for three smaller meals spread across their *eating window* instead of two meals a day. You can choose whatever works for you as long as you stay within your calorie budget. There is some evidence to suggest that eating a little earlier in the day benefitted people's metabolism, even in cases where there was no weight loss (Dady, 2021).

When it comes to food selection, the same advice given earlier still stands. Choose nutrient-dense foods that will give you high-quality proteins, high fiber, and plenty of essential vitamins and minerals. Fish, chicken, lean meat, yogurt, and eggs are the best sources of protein. Dark leafy vegetables and berries supply essential vitamins and fiber. Legumes and lentils will supply protein, fiber, and essential minerals. Don't forget to add healthy fats such as olive oil and avocados, and always hydrate with non-calorie drinks like tea, coffee, and water (still or sparkling). It's also a very good idea to supplement with a good multivitamin to boost your health and "increase energy levels, especially if it is rich in B vitamins" (Dady, 2021).

How Safe Is the 5:2 Method?

The 5:2 method is safe for most people and is an effective method to help you lose weight, as demonstrated by the studies cited here and elsewhere. However, it is still not recommended for the following groups of people:

- pregnant and breastfeeding mothers
- those who are trying to conceive
- those younger than 18 years
- those with a history of eating disorders
- people who are on medication
- people who are malnourished, underweight, or have nutrient deficiencies
- those who often experience drops in blood sugar levels

The Eat Stop Eat Method

The Eat Stop Eat (ESE) method gets its name from Brad Pilon, who wrote the book *Eat Stop Eat: The Shocking Truth That Makes Weight Loss Simple Again.* With this method, you also fast on one or two nonconsecutive days a week and eat normally on the five or six remaining days. The difference here, however, is that you should observe a complete 24-hour fast on your fasting days. Let's give an example. If your fast starts at 9 a.m. on a certain day of the week, say Tuesday or Wednesday, the next time you eat will be only once 24 hours are over, which will be after 9 a.m. the following day. Similar to the other methods, you are supposed to eat *freely* on the non-fasting days, but we have already discussed what this means for a disciplined intermittent faster who does not plan to go over their calorie allowance. Pilon also suggests that you boost your results by combining this method with a strength training plan. We have already mentioned some of the research that shows that combining IF with a training program has the potential to double your weight loss efforts.

The Benefits of the ESE Method

Fasting for 24 hours allows the body to go into *ketosis*, which we spoke about in the earlier chapters. Ketosis kicks in once the glycogen stores are depleted, and the body switches to burning fat. This is what we mean by *metabolic switching*. Your body starts making ketones at this stage, and these become your primary source of energy. This is also the point at which weight loss is triggered, and it is what makes this method so effective in producing weight reduction (Anton et al., 2018). I would like to caution here that not everyone reaches ketosis at the same time, and therefore, more data is required to understand the variability here.

Secondly, the overall calorie deficit that happens due to the 24-hour fast days on this method is one of the most obvious ways in which weight loss is triggered. When you don't eat for one or two days a week, you create a weekly calorie deficit that produces weight loss. The downside of this method is that not everyone can pull off a 24-hour fast. It is also likely to cause certain nutrient deficiencies for those who are not closely watching what they are eating on their non-fasting days to ensure that they eat a balanced diet. A balanced diet would give them all the required nutrients like proteins, carbohydrates, fats, vitamins, and minerals for the body to function well.

The ESE method has been used to improve blood sugar levels, and although most people have no problems maintaining healthy levels during fasting, some suggest that this method may not be suitable for those with diabetes because the extended fast may drop their blood sugar to even more dangerous levels. There is evidence to suggest that it may be safe and effective in populations that suffer from both type 1 and type 2 diabetes when done under the supervision of a healthcare provider with consistent glucose monitoring (Grajower & Horne, 2019).

What Do You Eat on the ESE Method?

Since you will be fasting for a full 24 hours, it is very important that you stay hydrated while fasting. Drink lots of water, tea, coffee, and low-calorie or *diet* drinks. You can also use artificial sweeteners in your tea and coffee. The ESE method, like other IF methods, does not have any specific requirements in terms of what to eat during your eating days, the main rule being that you completely abstain from eating for a full 24-hour period on your fasting days. It is still advisable that you do not overindulge on your eating days and that you try to limit your choices to the foods that will give you optimal nutrition for your body, as listed under the IF methods discussed above.

How Safe Is the ESE Method?

Because of the low blood sugar that may be experienced during fasting days, this method is generally not recommended for those who are on medications that lower blood sugar unless practiced under the supervision of a healthcare provider. It is also not recommended for those special populations that it hasn't been tested on, as listed under the other IF methods. The ESE method, like other IF methods, may contribute to hormonal changes in women, although some research shows positive changes, specifically for those who may suffer from polycystic ovary syndrome (PCOS) (Cienfuegos et al., 2022). There is mixed data. It would therefore be best for those who are trying to become pregnant to consult a physician before they start on this method. The ESE method is otherwise safe and effective for weight loss in healthy adults.

Time-Restricted Feeding

On TRF plans, IF is practiced on a daily basis, but you choose the number of hours you want to fast per day versus the number of hours you will be eating. So the schedules to choose from vary by length of *eating window* versus *fasting time*. The different schedules are presented below:

The Crescendo Fasting Method

Regarded by many as the best method for women, we will get into the reasons why a bit later on in this chapter. The Crescendo method is also one of the easiest and, therefore, more suitable for those who are new to IF. On this plan, you fast for two to three days a week as long as you make sure that those are nonconsecutive days. It is best to start two days a week until you get used to fasting and increase the days as you get more experienced. The name Crescendo is based on exactly that, the fact that it eases you into fasting by gently increasing the days and/or hours of fasting as you progress on your IF journey. On the fasting days, you would choose how many hours you fast versus how many hours you set aside as your *eating window*. As a newbie, you could perhaps start with a 12:12 plan, gently increasing your fasting window and shortening your eating window to a 16:8 plan as you get more comfortable with fasting. At this point, you may also want to consider increasing your fasting days to three days instead of two a week. We will look at the 16:8 method in detail in the next section.

What Are the Benefits of the Crescendo Fasting Method?

There isn't much research that has been dedicated to this method specifically, but just like the other IF methods, it is expected that the Crescendo method would carry the same benefits such as the ones listed below:

- *Insulin and type 2 diabetes*: A number of different studies have shown that IF could reduce insulin resistance and reverse type 2 diabetes. Some of those studies were presented in the first chapter, including a randomized clinical trial by Harvie et al. (2010).

- *Gut health*: Animal studies showed that IF improved gut health, starved gut bacteria, improved intolerances, and increased life expectancy (Catterson et al., 2018).
- *Improved fertility*: A review of both animal and human studies led to the conclusion that IF increases the release of luteinizing hormones in women suffering from PCOS (Nair & Khawale, 2016). This could directly promote ovulation in women.

Other health benefits of IF include decreased dangerous body fat, improved metabolism, and reduced inflammation.

What to Eat on the Crescendo Method?

First of all, stay hydrated. We've already discussed what this means on IF and the type of drinks to include. Hydration is important because your body loses a lot of water during fasting. As the glycogen stores get depleted, and insulin levels drop, your body excretes more sodium, which results in your body losing more water and getting dehydrated (Jockers, 2019). If you are one of those people who don't like the taste of plain water, you can add stevia to your water or lemon slices, depending on what you fancy. I also recommend that you add sea salt, especially in the initial stages, as your body loses electrolytes. Losing electrolytes show up as fatigue, light-headedness, confusion, and digestion issues.

There are no hard and fast rules when it comes to what foods to eat on this plan, just like in all the other IF plans, except the general guidelines to limit your choices to nutrient-dense foods that will provide your body with optimal health. Choose wholesome and organic foods, and try to stay away from refined carbohydrates and junk food. It is also recommended that you supplement with branched-chain amino acids (BCAAs). These are not naturally produced by the body, and that is why you should take them as supplements. BCAAs can help keep the hunger pangs at bay, with muscle building and decreasing fatigue, among other benefits.

Is the Crescendo Method Safe?

Even though all IF methods have been shown to be safe in healthy adults, and as much as the Crescendo method is the gentlest for beginners, it is still not for everyone. You are advised to stop if you don't feel well, if your cycle is disturbed, or if you are constantly feeling *rundown*. It would be best to consult your healthcare advisor at this point. It is also possible that these may just be teething problems as your body adjusts to a new way of eating, but it is always best to err on the side of caution.

This method is not recommended for those who have been diagnosed with eating disorders as it may trigger unhealthy eating patterns. It is not recommended for children, pregnant and lactating women, and those on other medications as it has not been tested on them and safety is not guaranteed for these populations.

The 16:8 Plan

This is one of the most popular plans as most people find it easier to stick to and fit into their lifestyles. The 16:8, as the name suggests, is where you fast for 16 hours and have an eight-hour eating window. Most people find this schedule easier because they can eat their meals during the daytime and fast overnight, starting in the late afternoon or early evening. For example, you could eat from 8 a.m. to 4 p.m. or from 10 a.m. to 6 p.m. You can pick any time slot really, depending on your lifestyle. If you know that you always have dinner engagements with family or friends, you can pick a later schedule that allows your eating window to end a little later in the day.

What Are the Benefits of this Method?

- *Weight loss*: The calorie deficit created by limiting your eating window results in less calorie intake, which leads to weight loss. Although most of these studies are not specific to each IF regime, a review of studies done by Patterson et al. (2015) showed that the TRF methods produced significant weight loss, with one study showing up to 4.1% weight loss in comparison to other methods.
- *Blood sugar control*: As discussed previously, IF has been shown to help control blood sugar due to the decreased number of meals, causing fewer insulin spikes. In the same review mentioned above, one study demonstrated that eating once a day, which is another version of TRF methods, resulted in both reductions in glucose levels and improvements in LDL and HDL cholesterol when compared to other diets.

Other studies have shown that it might contribute to longevity, and one way this is possible is through autophagy which was discussed in an earlier chapter, the process where the body gets rid of neurodegenerative cells.

What to Eat on This Plan?

The 16:8 plan does not specify which foods to eat, but caution should be exercised not to overindulge so as to stay within your calorie allowance and to stay within the foods that are nutrient-dense to provide optimal health for your body. One can use these guidelines to choose what to eat:

- high-quality protein sources: fish, lean meats, and high-quality dairy
- whole grains: quinoa, barley, brown rice, and oats
- fruits and vegetables: dark leafy vegetables and berries

- healthy fats: olive oil, coconuts, avocados, fatty fish, and nuts and seeds
- low- or zero-calorie drinks: tea, coffee, water, and diet drinks

The 20:4 or Warrior Diet

On this plan, you fast for 20 hours and eat over a four-hour window each day. This method is also known as the *Warrior Diet* and was created by Ori Hofmekler in 2001. It is called the *Warrior Diet* because it is loosely based on "the eating habits of ancient warriors who ate very little during the day and feasted at night" (Kubala, 2018). This method is not based on science, as the founder, Hofmekler himself has admitted that it is based on his own beliefs and observations.

What Are the Benefits of This Plan?

Research has not been done specifically on this plan, but it is expected that it would carry similar benefits to other IF plans. In a study that employed a similar regimen, those who ate only one meal a day showed a significant reduction in fat mass and improved muscle mass (Stote et al., 2007). A concern voiced for those who embark on this plan is that they may go over their daily calorie allowance by binging during the short eating window, thus negating the effects of IF.

Secondly, this plan may contribute to reduced inflammation due to the combined effects of the reduced number of eating episodes and the process of autophagy. Similar results were observed in a 16:8 study, where there were significant reductions in levels of *tumor necrosis factor alpha (TNF-α)* and *interleukin-1 beta (IL-1β)* (Moro et al., 2016). These are the substances that promote inflammation. Inflammation has a direct link to diseases like heart disease, diabetes, and some cancers.

This plan may also contribute to brain health because of reduced inflammation. Studies in animals showed a reduction in inflammation markers such as *IL-6* and *TNF-α* (Shojaie et al., 2017). These negatively impact memory and learning.

The third benefit of this plan is blood sugar control. Fasting for 18–20 hours was shown to lead to a significant decrease in weight and improved fasting and post-meal blood sugar in those with type 2 diabetes (Arnason et al., 2017).

So What Does One Eat on This Method?

According to Hofmekler, dieters can consume small amounts of healthy nuts and seeds, dairy, hard-boiled or poached eggs, fruits, and vegetables, as well as low-calorie drinks during the fasting window, but they can eat as much as they like during the four-hour eating window. He does, however, caution that dieters should try to eat as much healthy, unprocessed, and organic food as possible during this window.

There is a suggested three-week plan for those who are starting on this plan to help them kick-start their IF journey, and it is presented below:

Week 1 is called the *detox week*: Here, you are encouraged to eat small portions of the following: vegetable juice, clear vegetable broth, poached or hard-boiled eggs, dairy (could be cottage cheese or yogurt), and fruits and vegetables (raw) during the fasting window, and *overeat* on salads with healthy oil and vinegar, to be followed up a bit later with a large meal or two medium-sized meals made of plant proteins, whole grains, small amounts of cheese, and vegetables (cooked). You can drink as much as you like of the zero- or low-calorie drinks (black coffee, tea, seltzer, diet drinks, and water).

Week 2 is a *high-fat week*: During this week, you are encouraged to follow the same protocol as week 1 during your fasting hours.

During your eating hours, you are encouraged to choose from a salad made with healthy oil and vinegar, followed up with a lean protein and cooked vegetables, and you can introduce a handful of nuts. You should not consume any grains and/or starches in week 2. Keep your eye on your hydration with zero- or low-calorie drinks.

Week 3 is called the *concluding fat loss*. At this stage, you will cycle between periods of high-carb and high-protein or low-carb intake. The periods of high-carb versus high-protein intake can be one to two days on each, on a rotation.

On **high-carb** days, you should eat as per protocol for fasting hours, meaning small amounts of eggs (hard-boiled or poached), dairy, raw fruits and vegetables, broth, and vegetable juice. During the eating window, you will eat a salad with healthy oil and vinegar and put together a meal or two made up of small amounts of animal protein and cooked vegetables, and you can have one main carb such as pasta, barley, potatoes, corn, oats, etc.

On **high-protein, low-carb days**, this is how you should eat: Eat small amounts of clear vegetable broth, vegetable juices, hard-boiled or poached eggs, dairy (this could be yogurt or cottage cheese), and fruits and vegetables (raw). During the eating window, you should eat as above but also include about 8–16 oz of animal proteins and a side of cooked non-starchy vegetables. A small amount of tropical fruit may also be added here, but I caution you not to indulge in starches and/or grains in this phase. You may do this if you feel like adding a *dessert* to your meal.

It is also recommended that you add a multivitamin, probiotics, and amino acids here to supplement your diet. According to Hofmekler, one should then cycle back to the beginning (week 1) once week 3 is completed, and you can keep doing this for as long as possible. Should you not want to do that, the general advice is to just eat small portions of the low-calorie foods suggested for the fasting window and choose from the foods suggested for the eating window. You must do this while making sure that you add protein-rich meals during the eating window and minimizing the starch and carbs as much as possible.

Are TRF Methods Safe?

Generally considered safe for healthy adults, TRF methods are not suitable for people who are at risk of eating disorders as they may trigger those conditions. These plans are also not suitable for women who are trying to conceive, are pregnant, or breastfeeding (Leonard, 2020). It may also not be suitable for those who suffer from depression and anxiety, although there is some research that suggests that short-term calorie restriction may alleviate these conditions (Zhang et al., 2015).

Those who already live with diabetes are also cautioned to consult with their healthcare provider before embarking on this plan to assess their suitability for this method. This plan is also not suitable for the groups of people that it has not been tested on: children and those who are on certain medications. You are advised to speak to your doctor if you are not sure if you would be the right candidate for it.

The Warrior Diet specifically may not be for everyone, and caution is advised. Some of the potential side effects that have been identified are the following (Harvie & Howell, 2017):

- fatigue
- dizziness
- low energy
- insomnia
- light-headedness
- low blood sugar
- hormonal imbalance
- irritability
- constipation

- extreme hunger
- weight gain

So Which Plan Is Best for Women?

Because IF impacts women's and men's health differently, as discussed in previous chapters, with reproductive hormones affected, as shown in lab studies with rats, it is advisable that women choose IF plans that have shorter fasting periods or those with fewer fasting days than the opposite. One study showed that mice who were on ADF for three to six months had a reduction in the size of their ovaries and had irregular reproductive cycles (Kumar & Kaur, 2013). This may be a concern, especially for those who still want to have children. IF has also been associated with a reduction in the hormone estrogen, which would negatively impact a woman's ability to conceive. Scientists think this is because of the hormone kisspeptin, a hormone that is responsible for the production of male and female sex hormones, testosterone and estrogen. IF decreases kisspeptin leading to infertility and amenorrhea (Mudge, 2022). It is not only the reproductive hormones that are affected by IF. Another study showed that blood sugar level control got worse after 22 days on the ADF plan for women than men (Heilbronn, Civitarese, et al., 2005).

Bearing all of the above in mind, it is recommended that women choose plans that support their health rather than those that might have an adverse effect on their health.

Some of the plans that have been identified as best for women are the following:

- *The Crescendo fasting method*: This method has been identified as potentially the best IF method for women because unlike the other methods that have you fasting for anywhere between 12 and 20 hours, this one cuts the fasting time to just 12–16 hours only twice or three times a week.

This happens on nonconsecutive days. Choosing the Crescendo method also allows your body plenty of time to get accustomed to fasting without adding unnecessary stress to the sudden change of going without food. As you get better at fasting, you can then switch to the other IF methods with longer fasting hours, such as the 16:8 ("Crescendo Fasting," 2022). In this way, this method is a great stepping stone to introducing you and getting your body ready for the other IF plans.

The Crescendo method also helps you not to develop bad eating habits because of how it is structured. The other reason this may be the best method for women is that restricting your calorie intake has the potential to negatively impact your menstrual cycle, but with the Crescendo method, the calorie intake is not severely restricted, which allows the emphasis not to be so much on calorie restriction but rather on eating at certain hours to optimize hormones for weight loss. Crescendo fasting also allows you the flexibility to combine your diet with strength training on non-fasting days, which gives an additional boost to your weight loss efforts.

- *The 16:8 method*: This plan may be better suited for women as it can also be modified where you can start with a shorter fasting window, such as a 14-hour window, and extend as you get more comfortable. It also allows the flexibility of scheduling your meals later in the day so that if you are a mom who wants to enjoy her meals with the family, you can easily do that. In other words, it is adaptable to and suitable for different lifestyles.
- *The modified ADF*: On this plan, you will have to consume at least 500 calories of food on your fasting days and eat *normally* on the non-fasting days. You also have to make sure that you allow at least one day between your fasting

days and that you do not do more than two fasting days a week.

- *The 5:2 plan*: The first thing to ensure if you choose this plan is that you do not observe more than two days of fasting a week on it. Adapt the plan by making sure that you eat 500 calories of your daily allowance on your fasting days instead of going for a complete 24-hour fast.
- *Eat Stop Eat plan*: This plan is made up of one to two days of 24-hour fasting, but for women, you can adapt it by doing shorter fasts of 14–16 hours at a time on your fasting days. Once you get comfortable with fasting, you can gradually extend your fasts to 24 hours.

Now that we have explained how each of the plans works, which plan do you think would be best for you? The different plans offer almost the same benefits in terms of weight loss, insulin regulation, disease prevention, lessened inflammation, etc., so you would just have to think about your lifestyle mainly and decide what would work best for you. If you are still not sure, especially if you are on any medications, please seek the counsel of your doctor.

Chapter 4: Intermittent Fasting After 50

What Are the Benefits of Intermittent Fasting for Pre and Postmenopausal Women?

Women encounter many health issues in their pre and postmenopausal phase of life, and many have no choice but to start taking various medications to manage these conditions. In this chapter, we are going to discuss how IF can serve as a healthy alternative, a non-pharmacological *therapy* that addresses some of these health conditions.

Cancer Risk

One of the main health conditions prevalent at this stage of life is cancer. Cancer is the leading cause of morbidity and mortality, with approximately 20 million new cases and 10 million deaths reported in 2020 (World Health Organization, 2022). Among women, the most common cancers are breast, colorectum, lung, cervix, and stomach cancer, with breast cancer being regarded as the second most common in the world and leading among women. The WHO lists an unhealthy diet, which results in a high BMI, among the top five risk factors for cancer. What this tells us is that some of these conditions are preventable.

Weight gain is a health concern that features as a big concern for women over 50 for various reasons. Women over 50 tend to pick up weight easily due to a slowed-down metabolism and achy joints, which leads to a reduction in physical activity, and even irregular sleep. Since aging also contributes to a loss in lean muscle, lean muscle is linked to a faster metabolism; it makes sense then that as women age, they start losing that lean muscle and, as a result, gain weight easily. We also start seeing increased abdominal fat in this age group. Extra belly fat is not just a concern for aesthetics, but it has been scientifically linked to diseases such as heart disease, cholesterol, type 2 diabetes, high blood pressure, and some cancers, as stated above.

So how can IF address these health concerns? In a systematic review of studies done in 2016, the researchers concluded that IF could play a significant role in protecting people against cancer. In their words, "fasting can theoretically inhibit several critical pathways in the development and progression of cancer while simultaneously causing malignancies more sensitive to treatments, for instance, chemotherapy and radiotherapy" (Nair & Khawale, 2016). Another study demonstrated that in mice with breast cancer, fasting for 48 hours significantly suppressed the growth of the tumor (Lee et al., 2012).

Metabolic Health

A number of cardiovascular diseases (CVDs) that appear together or coexist in a person are referred to as a syndrome of CVD and diabetes. Although this syndrome tends to present years later in women than in men, it usually shows a marked increase in menopausal women. Some of these risk factors are increased belly fat, increased LDL and triglyceride levels, decreased HDL levels, and increased glucose and insulin levels. Various studies, and most recently, one done by Varady et al. (2021), have shown that IF protects against CVDs. This study showed results of weight loss, reduction of fat tissue mass, decreased blood pressure and heart rate, and a decrease in total cholesterol and LDL cholesterol levels, as well as an increase in HDL cholesterol levels after the subjects were put on different IF regimens.

Heart health is very important for women in this age group. The research cited above shows the great benefits of IF in protecting your heart's health by lessening all the risk factors that we've listed above. More recent confirmation came from a randomized control trial that showed that IF could protect the heart by increasing the production of a key protein that controls inflammation (Bartholomew et al., 2021).

A study that compared three groups of people with obesity—premenopausal women, postmenopausal women, and men—followed them over a period of 12 weeks on the ADF regimen to see if its weight loss efficacy differs by gender. The results showed similar reductions in fat mass, lean mass, fasting insulin, insulin resistance, and blood pressure across all three groups. What should be of great interest to a woman 50 years and older is that in that study, postmenopausal women showed greater declines in LDL cholesterol compared to premenopausal women (Lin et al., 2020).

Another study that compared pre and postmenopausal women with obesity using TRF methods showed similar results in weight loss and improvements in the metabolism across both groups (Cienfuegos et al., 2021). This, too, is good news for postmenopausal women who experience additional challenges when it comes to weight loss at their age. These are exacerbated by hormonal changes that result in a decline in estrogen, leaving them at increased risk for weight gain, CVDs, and many issues with regulating blood sugar levels.

Other hormonal changes that take place at this age are an increase in cortisol, thyroid hormones, serotonin, and sex hormones which become negatively affected. As a woman, if you experience compromised insulin sensitivity during menopause, this may leave you less able to process sugar and refined carbohydrates. When this happens, it translates directly to weight gain, especially around the midsection. But we know now that IF helps to *flip the metabolic switch*, and it does this by helping the body produce less insulin when you fast. Less insulin means less glycogen stored in the body, and this helps the body to burn the fat that is already stored in your body.

Four weeks of fasting has been shown to reduce BMI, weight, and waist circumference (Sadiya et al., 2011). This signifies the role of IF in fighting metabolic diseases that are most common in older women. In this way, IF is a great weight loss tool for women over 50.

Mental Health

Menopausal women experience a lot of mental issues due to the life transition that they are going through. About 80%–85% of women struggle with some of the unpleasant menopausal symptoms they experience during this transition (Elavsky & McAuley, 2007). Some of the most common symptoms are night sweats, hot flashes, moodiness, anxiety, irritability, and even emotional instability. The role of IF in alleviating some mental health conditions, such as depression and anxiety, has been well documented (Koushali et al., 2013), albeit in different populations.

IF may decrease susceptibility to anxiety and depression and, according to WebMD, the emotional roller coaster that sometimes accompanies hormonal changes during menopause (Brennan, 2021).

In earlier chapters, we also spoke about how IF improves cognitive function by triggering the production of *brain-derived neurotrophic factor* (BDNF), a hormone that improves concentration and mental flexibility. Studies have shown that low amounts of BDNF are linked to poor brain health and, in some cases, depression. Since IF also reduces the risk for neurodegenerative diseases such as Alzheimer's and Parkinson's through autophagy, it has become very evident how this diet is beneficial for women during this phase of life.

Musculoskeletal Health

Musculoskeletal conditions affect millions of people around the world and are a cause of pain and physical disability to many. They also affect the psychosocial status of those affected. These conditions can show up as early onset, short-lived, or life-long conditions, and unfortunately, their presence increases with age. Here, we are talking about conditions such as osteoporosis, arthritis, and lower back pain. These are some of the conditions you may start to experience as you advance in age.

Can IF help in preventing these conditions? The answer is *yes*. Research has shown that IF is good for improving bone health. Fasting for 7–10 days reduced stiffness, pain, and dependency on analgesics significantly in patients with rheumatoid arthritis (Sköldstam et al., 1979). This confirms the role of IF in preventing inflammation, a major contributing factor to musculoskeletal disorders. As one grows older, conditions like osteoporosis start showing up due to the decreasing bone mineral density. IF slows the progressions of these age-related conditions. Secondly, since fasting helps in the reduction of body weight, it therefore, helps in reducing the risk of fractures and other similar conditions.

IF has other benefits, such as tissue health and increased physical performance, that have been reported anecdotally, and so overall, it's a great disease prevention tool for women in their 50s and above.

Chapter 5: What to Eat on Intermittent Fasting

We have spoken at length about the health benefits of doing IF, and hopefully, by now, we have helped you select the best method for you, depending on your health concerns and your lifestyle, of course.

In this next chapter, we will delve a bit deeper into what to eat while you are IF to equip you with the right tools to ensure your success.

The big question is, *can you eat whatever you like on IF?* Most people seem to think so, but this is not true, as you may have realized this by now just by going through the first four chapters of this book. So then, what to eat? A healthy and varied diet will be key to your success on this journey. It has to be *healthy* because that is the whole point of doing IF, to adopt a healthy eating lifestyle, but also *varied* because you don't want to get bored by eating the same foods over and over. That is a surefire way to quickly lose interest and return to your old unhealthy habits. The other important reason for eating a healthy diet is that when you do so, you are feeding the bacteria that live inside your gut the nutrients that it requires in order to maintain the healthy functioning of your body.

So the best thing you can do for yourself before you start on the IF plan that you have selected is to go out and purchase the best-quality foods to fill your cupboard with and get rid of junk food as much as possible. Discipline is going to be your key to success on this journey.

What Do We Mean by *Good-Quality Foods*?

Good-quality or high-quality food is food that provides your body with the fiber, protein, vitamins, and minerals that it requires to function properly *and* also keep you full for longer so you can avoid irresponsible snacking.

Here, I'm going to spend a bit of time talking about a group of foods called *superfoods*. You may have heard of the term *superfoods*, but do you know what those are and why they are called *superfoods*? Let me start by answering the second part of the question before providing a list of these types of food. If you perform a search of the meaning of the term *superfoods* on Google, you will quickly learn, from reliable sources, that this term was started as a marketing gimmick. There is no such thing as a superfood, not according to science anyway. In 2007, the EU went as far as banning the term from being attached to food labels if there was no scientific evidence that this was the case. However, between 2011 and 2015, there was a huge spike in global sales of foods that were marketed as *superfoods*. According to the Mintel Global New Products Database, this spike was a 202% increase in the sales of food and drinks containing the label *superfood, superfruit,* and *supergrain* (Mintel Press Team, 2016).

So why call any food or drink a *superfood* anyway, and why do we still continue to use this term when talking about certain foods? This is because there are certain foods, based on their superior nutritional content, that have earned this label from the healthy lifestyle community. These are basically the types of food that deliver the best nutrition for your body. As a sidenote, because of the huge demand from consumers for the best products, which is happening because people are becoming more health conscious, we are starting to see the term *super* being applied to other consumer products such as beauty and other health products, as well as pet food, etc.

So What Foods Fall Under the Label of "Superfood"?

According to Migala (2020), the banana may have been the first fruit to ever receive this label, and this can be traced back to over a century ago, when research commissioned by the United Fruit Company in 1920 touted the health benefits of a banana, resulting in the fruit gaining much popularity and being called a superfood. Bananas are still among the top three most imported fruits in the US (Brooks, 2020).

Berries

Berries are packed with vitamins, minerals, and fiber, as well as antioxidants. In previous chapters, we spoke about the role of antioxidants in reducing the risk of certain cancers, heart disease, and even some inflammatory conditions. A review of nutrition studies showed that berries may be effective at treating digestive and immune-related disorders, as well as in the reduction of the number and size of premalignant and malignant lesions (Govers et al., 2017). Now, you can understand why this fruit deserves to be called a superfood.

Berries may also help to keep you mentally sharp because they have anthocyanidins. In a study where researchers reviewed data from over 16,000 women over the age of 70, they concluded that eating a serving of blueberries or two servings of strawberries a week showed less mental decline over time (Devore et al., 2012). Berries may help reduce your risk of diabetes too. A study that followed 500,000 Chinese adults showed that those who consumed fresh fruit daily were 12% less likely to develop diabetes (Du et al., 2017), and since berries are also lower on the glycemic index, they are the best choice for managing your blood sugar levels.

The best thing about berries is the fact that they are one of the best-tasting fruits and are so versatile. They can easily be added to your smoothies and breakfasts, such as oatmeal and salads, and make a great snack instead of candy.

Avocado

The health benefits of avocados are widely publicized, which is why this fruit also earns a place in the *superfoods* category. They are packed with vitamins, minerals, and fiber. Half an avocado provides the body with 29 mg of magnesium (USDA, 2019), which plays a big role in regulating blood pressure, blood sugar, and magnesium deficiency. A magnesium deficiency puts you at risk of type 2 diabetes. Research also shows that avocados may reduce your risk of getting metabolic syndrome, heart diseases, certain types of cancers, and diabetes (Fulgoni et al., 2013).

Most people fear avocados because they have high-calorie content, but what most don't understand is that, even though this is the case, avocados are packed with what we call *good fats*, also known as *unsaturated* fats. Why is that a good thing, you may wonder? Unsaturated fats help lower one's LDL cholesterol levels in the body and reduce inflammation. Avocados contain what is called oleic acid, a monounsaturated fat that has been proven scientifically to fight inflammation in your body (Sales-Campos et al., 2013).

Avocados also help to keep you full for longer so you don't overeat when you include them in your diet. They are also easy to add to your diet, and you can do this by adding them to salads or just spreading them onto your toast.

Whole grains

Whole grains deliver the best nutrients because they have *not* been stripped of the outer layer, called *bran*, which is rich in fiber and has B vitamins, iron, copper, zinc, magnesium, antioxidants, and phytochemicals (Harvard T.H. Chan School of Public Health, 2018). Phytochemicals fight off diseases. The *germ*, the smallest part inside the kernel, provides the body with vitamin E, B vitamins, phytochemicals, and antioxidants. If you compare that to the *endosperm*, the inner part that refined grains are made of, it only gives us carbohydrates, protein, minerals, and small amounts of B vitamins.

So the best thing to do when it comes to this food group is to pick those grains that are unrefined over their refined counterparts. So instead of eating white rice, you should consider substituting it with brown rice. A study published in 2018 reported that brown rice contains a variety of phenolic acids, and these have antioxidant properties that lessen your risk of type 2 diabetes, cancer, and heart disease (Ravichanthiran et al., 2018).

Other good grains to choose from are bulgur wheat, barley, and oats. According to Harvard T.H. Chan School of Public Health (2018), these grains are packed with fiber, vitamins, and antioxidants. You may also be aware of the new buzzword in health circles with regard to grains, and that is *ancient grains*. Ancient grains are now the new superfood, but according to the Whole Grains Council, they are referred to as *ancient grains* simply because nothing has changed with regard to how these foods were produced a hundred years ago. In other words, they have maintained their *innocence*. Those grains are quinoa, buckwheat, and farro.

Vegetables

The dark leafy vegetables are always the best in terms of nutrition, providing us with fiber, vitamin C, zinc, calcium, iron, magnesium, and folate. The darker the green color, the more nutrient-dense the vegetable is. The American Institute for Cancer Research (2020) lists vegetables like kale, for instance, as one of those with powerful antioxidants that may prevent the formation of carcinogens. These may be effective in preventing cancers like colorectal cancer. Another class of vegetables that you should definitely consider is *cruciferous* vegetables. Cauliflower, broccoli, and brussels sprouts are all cruciferous vegetables. They are rich in fiber which means they keep you full for longer and regular. Broccoli may also prevent breast cancer. One study showed that broccoli contains sulforaphane, a compound that reduces the cancer stem cell markers in 65%–80% of human breast cancer cells (Li et al., 2010).

So the choice is wide, when it comes to vegetables to choose from to include in your diet. Consider adding broccoli, spinach, collard greens, kale, Swiss chard, and turnip greens. These vegetables are also the best source of carotenoids, anti-inflammatory compounds that may protect you from some types of cancers (Xavier & Pérez-Gálvez, 2016). Research has shown that vegetables may lower your risk for heart disease and other chronic illnesses (Blekkenhorst et al., 2018) and diabetes (Wang et al., 2015).

Vegetables are good for stews and soups in winter and salads in summer. You can also stir-fry them or add them to your smoothies.

Nuts and Seeds

Packed with fiber, vegetarian protein, and healthy fats, nuts and seeds are great for vegetarians who don't get their protein from animal sources. Almonds are good for heart health, whereas cashews are great for brain power, and Brazil nuts have been praised for cancer prevention. Harvard reports on some research that shows that those who regularly eat nuts are less likely to suffer from heart attacks than those who don't. This is based on studies that show a 30%–50% lower risk of myocardial infarction, sudden death, or cardiovascular diseases (Harvard T.H. Chan School of Public Health, 2012). Scientists think this is due to the unsaturated fats that lower the LDL and raise the HDL cholesterol. The same report makes an example of walnuts which contain omega-3 fatty acids that prevent the development of erratic heart rhythms and also prevent blood clots. Nuts also keep you full for longer, which ultimately helps you eat less. In this way, they prevent weight gain and obesity, a great reason for adding them to your IF lifestyle. Nuts may also lower your risk of type 2 diabetes, according to a study that concluded that those who ate a serving of 28 grams of nuts per week had a 17% lower risk of cardiovascular diseases (Harvard T.H. Chan School of Public Health, 2012).

Seeds are, on the other hand, packed with vitamins and minerals. Good examples of seeds are hemp, chia, and flaxseeds. You can add these onto your smoothies or sprinkle over your salad.

Protein

Great sources of protein include eggs, fish, poultry, steak, cottage cheese, natural yogurt, plain kefir, legumes, nuts and seeds, and protein powders. Just make sure to avoid the ones with sugar added. Tofu is also a good source of protein for those who don't eat meat.

Eggs

Eggs have truly earned the label of a superfood, and that is because they are packed with vitamin A, B vitamins, iron, phosphorus, choline, and selenium, and one large egg gives you 6.24 g of protein. Eggs also contain two very powerful antioxidants named zeaxanthin and lutein. Those who are concerned about the high cholesterol content should know that it has been shown, through research, that there is no correlation between eating eggs and having high cholesterol. This was tested on people who had up to 12 eggs a week (Richard et al., 2017). Another study confirmed that eggs increased

HDL, the good cholesterol, and this may reduce your risk of cardiovascular diseases (Blesso & Luz Fernandez, 2018).

We also love the versatility of eggs because as much as they are *breakfast food,* they can be prepared in so many different ways and can be added to salads as well. Eggs also keep you full for longer, another great benefit for fasters.

Fish and Seafood

Seafood is a great source of protein, vitamin D, and healthy fats, especially fatty fish such as salmon. Salmon and sardines are high in omega-3 fatty acids. A 100 g of wild Atlantic salmon has 2.2 g of omega-3s, high-quality animal protein, magnesium, potassium, selenium, and B vitamins (USDA, 2019). Always try to choose the wild salmon instead of the farmed variant. It contains a better omega-6 to omega-3 ratio and fewer contaminants. An imbalance of omega-6 and omega-3 in your body may lead to certain chronic diseases.

Shellfish is more nutritious as it comes with vitamin C, various B vitamins, potassium, selenium, and iron. A hundred grams of clams contain 16 times the Recommended Dietary Intake (RDI) for vitamin B12. A hundred grams of oysters contain 600% of the RDI for zinc, 200% of the RDI for copper, and large amounts of vitamin D, vitamin B12, as well as other nutrients (USDA, 2019).

Adding at least two portions of seafood to your diet weekly may lower your risk of heart disease, dementia, and depression (Wang et al., 2006).

Beans and Legumes

One of the best things about legumes, also called pulses, is that they are an inexpensive, low glycemic index food that is a source of proteins, vitamins, carbohydrates, and fiber. They are a great protein source for people who do not eat meat too. Some of the popular ones are chickpeas, lentils, kidney beans, black beans, pinto beans, and peas. Legumes may play a role in the management of type 2 diabetes, reducing blood pressure and cholesterol (Mudryj et al., 2014). Pulses keep you full for longer too, and you can easily add them to soups and stews.

Probiotics

These are the little critters that live in your gut and whose job is to keep your microbiome (gut) happy. Basically, they are live microorganisms found in fermented foods like yogurt, kombucha, kefir, and sauerkraut, and they are also available as supplements. When your gut is not happy, you may experience problems like constipation (Rizzo, 2022). A happy gut is one with a good balance of good and bad bacteria because both types of bacteria perform different functions in the body.

Herbs and Spices

Other than the obvious function of making our food taste great, herbs and spices contain powerful anti-inflammatory properties and have almost no calories, so you should feel good about adding them to your meals. Some of the herbs and spices worth mentioning here are the following:

- *Sage* can improve brain function and memory, especially for those who have Alzheimer's disease.
- *Thyme* contains antibacterial and antifungal chemicals and has been used to treat coughs and alopecia (hair loss).
- *Rosemary* can prevent allergies and can help alleviate nasal congestion.
- *Cayenne pepper* contains capsaicin which helps to reduce appetite and could protect against certain cancers.
- *Ginger* has anti-inflammatory properties and can treat nausea.

- *Garlic* may improve heart health by reducing LDL cholesterol.
- *Turmeric* contains curcumin which has anti-inflammatory properties and may prevent heart diseases by improving blood flow.
- *Cinnamon* lowers blood sugar levels.
- *Cumin* may help with facilitating digestion and with reducing the symptoms of IBS.
- *Cardamom* may help reduce blood pressure among those who have high levels and may also protect against *Helicobacter pylori*, a bacterium that is a common cause of stomach ulcers (Mahady et al., 2005).

What About Beverages?

We have spoken at length about beverages in the previous chapters, but it is still worth mentioning those beverages that can be included in an IF plan here. The general guideline is to choose zero or low-calorie beverages such as black coffee, tea (many variants to choose from, mostly herbal), water (not the artificially sweetened type), and diet drinks (just be sure to always watch the calorie content).

The above list of foods is provided to help you make the best selections for your meal planning and shopping by helping you understand which foods are nutrient-dense and deliver the best health benefits for your body.

The other way to go about choosing the foods to incorporate into your diet is to go back to your reasons for wanting to do IF because that would be your best guide for choosing the foods that would provide for those needs. Below are two of the most common reasons people start IF, and depending on what yours are, you may rather prefer to base your choices on your reasons.

Eating for Heart Health

If your goal is to eat for heart health, consider adding foods that contain fiber and healthy fats to your diet, and watch your salt intake. These foods are the following:

- whole grains such as brown rice, quinoa, oatmeal, and other whole grains
- avocado oil, olive oil, nut butters, medium-chain triglycerides (MCTs), ghee, and olives
- fruits and vegetables, mostly the dark leafy types *and* avocados and berries
- nuts and seeds
- salmon, sardines, and shellfish, mainly those that provide omega-3s
- salt-free seasoning

Eating to Lower Inflammation

If your goal is to lower inflammation, focus on controlling unhealthy blood fat and sugar responses, and choose from these foods to add to your diet:

- foods high in anti-inflammatory properties that contain polyphenols and carotenoids, such as fruits and vegetables
- whole grains because they have powerful antioxidants and phytochemicals
- avocados
- eggs
- foods that are high in omega-3 fatty acids, like fish, seeds, and nuts

For more information on the anti-inflammatory diet, consider purchasing my other book, *The Anti-Inflammatory Diet Made*

Simple: A Complete Beginners' Guide with the Top 13 Anti-Inflammatory Foods and Tasty Cookbook Recipes by Gabriel Baker

What Not to Eat on the IF diet?

Having spoken at length about what foods to eat for optimum health on the IF plan, we should also mention those foods *not* to eat. This is by no means to say that if you eat these foods, anything catastrophic will happen to you, but remember, the whole aim of getting on IF is to eat as healthily as possible *and* to develop a healthy relationship with food. So if you do have something not strictly on the superfoods or nutrient-dense foods, don't beat yourself up about it. Vow to do better next time, or put in some extra time at the gym to burn the extra calories consumed.

Naturally, these are the foods I would advise against consuming or ask that you limit as much as possible:

- crackers
- pretzels
- crisps or chips
- cookies and cakes
- candies
- fruit juices
- sugary cereals
- highly sweetened drinks, including teas and coffees

Supplements

Let's talk about supplements before we end this section. Supplements are a great way to supplement the nutrients that your body is not getting from your diet. There could be concerns that when you are IF you may not be getting all the nutrients from your diet. IF itself should not cause any nutritional deficiencies because IF is not only about *what* you eat but also *when* you eat. However, it could happen that the eating plan you choose is low in vitamins and minerals, and not including electrolytes, micronutrients, and fatty acids to your diet could further hamper your healthy eating efforts. If this is the case, you should add supplements. Also, for people who are vegans or vegetarians, their food may not completely provide all the required nutrients to meet the body's daily needs, so supplementing is an excellent idea.

If you are concerned that supplements will break your fast, just make sure that you don't take them during the fasting window unless this is a specific requirement. Many supplements can be taken with food, and some, like zinc, may upset your tummy if taken on an empty stomach. So make sure to read the information leaflet, so you know when is the best time to take each supplement. The information on the leaflet will also tell you if the supplement contains artificial sweeteners and other empty calories or, even worse, if they are likely to further decrease your glucose levels. Some of the ones to watch out for that decrease glucose levels are chromium picolinate, berberine, and psyllium husk. Even though there is a long list of those that can be taken with food, below we provide a list of those that *should* be taken on an empty stomach:

- probiotics
- folic acid
- water-soluble vitamins, such as B and C
- iron
- tyrosine

There are no supplements that are specifically for people who do IF; however, the following are recommended for IF as they help with ketosis and other processes (Trumpfeller, 2020):

- *Omega-3 fatty acids* help with appetite suppression.

- *MCTs* assist with metabolism.
- *Curcumin* may decrease insulin resistance.
- *Soluble fiber* increases feelings of fullness (satiety) to keep you full for longer.

Please consult your doctor before you start taking supplements, as they would be in the best position to assess your needs.

Chapter 6: Let's Get Started

Now that you have all the information you need to understand how IF works, are you ready to start your IF journey? If so, this chapter will help you prepare by sharing some of the tools and strategies you will need to adopt as you get started on IF. Let's dive in.

Define Your Reasons and Set Your Goals

Define your reasons for wanting to start IF. Everyone will have a different reason for doing IF. It's very important to define your reason because that will be the motivation that keeps you going even when you are facing challenges. Some people may want to fast for reasons other than weight loss. It's important, therefore, to know upfront what your reasons are, as this will determine your course of action. If you are one of those people who is fasting for reasons other than weight loss, you may still want to maintain your weight. So this brings up the issue of calories consumed per day. So the first thing to do would be to figure out what your calorie needs are per day based on your goal. There are free online tools to help you figure this out depending on your activity level, sex, age, height, etc., such as this one: www.calculator.net/calorie-calculator.html.

Knowing your calorie allowance will help you to keep an eye on how much food you consume so that you don't end up going over your allowance unintentionally and end up gaining weight or not losing any if that is your goal.

Which Plan Are You Going to Try?

One of the biggest decisions you have to make is to decide which plan you are going to get on and how you are going to structure that to fit in with your lifestyle. If you are completely new to IF, you may choose to start on the Crescendo plan. On this plan, you could, for instance, decide to start on the 12:12 schedule over two days a week. As you get better at fasting, you will increase the number of hours and the number of days that you are fasting. If you are planning to try other methods, the advice I would give you is that you try one plan for a month at the very least before you move on to another plan. This will give you enough time to see if it works for you or not.

Exercise

The next question you should ask yourself is whether you are going to include a training program to boost your weight loss efforts or not. We discuss the benefits of combining exercise with IF in Chapter 7, but one of the most important questions raised is when is the best time to exercise? So once you have decided that you are going to add exercise, you need to ask yourself what time of the day will you dedicate to exercise? Lots of research supports exercising in the morning; however, this may not be suitable for everyone, and you are the only one who knows, depending on your lifestyle, which would be best for you. The type of exercise you choose will also depend on the type of IF plan that you choose. This too is covered in detail in the next chapter.

Having the Right Mindset

Beginning with the right mindset sets you up for success and will take you far on this journey. That is why we said, "Know your reasons for doing this," because those will be your biggest motivation. I am against the *all-or-nothing* approach, and by this, I mean be gentle with yourself; making one mistake shouldn't mean ditching the diet. Count your gains and not your losses. Celebrate the small wins, and if celebrating means allowing yourself to eat a slice of pizza, then do it. Just don't overdo it.

It's also important to remember that if you gained weight, this happened over time, years for some, and you should, therefore, not expect to lose it all in a few weeks. While we are on that subject, also remember that sometimes weight loss does not show on the scale but rather on how your clothes fit. Those who do weight training will know that when you gain muscle through strength training, this shows up as *weight* on the scale, and to an untrained eye, that can be scary, to say the least. A knowledgeable person understands that this doesn't mean that they have gained *fat*, especially if they can see the difference in the mirror or in how their clothes fit.

Figuring Out a Meal Plan and Stocking up on Essentials

Now that you know what IF plan you are getting on and whether you will be exercising or not, the next thing to do is to figure out some kind of meal plan that you are going to follow and then fill up your grocery cupboard with the essentials. It is always a good idea to plan your meals in advance for the week, at the least, so that when you go shopping, you have a list of what you will need for your meal preparation. If you need help with meal planning, consider using the tool provided by the Centers for Disease Control and Prevention (CDC) website called *MyPlate Plan*. This tool helps you see your daily food group targets and how much to eat to stay within your calorie allowance. You can access this tool from this link: www.myplate.gov/myplate-plan.

Meal planning helps to make sure that you don't find yourself reaching for the closest thing that's available, even if it's not good for you, just because you are too hungry to put together a decent meal. The saying, "when you fail to plan, you plan to fail," is true for this very reason.

When you go shopping, make sure that you choose a variety of good-quality complex carbohydrates, high-quality protein, fresh fruit, and a lot of dark green leafy vegetables, as well as good fats. We covered this in Chapter 5. If you are going to need snacks, you also have to make sure that those are wholesome and not sugar-laden types of *nutrition* bars and energy drinks. While on the subject of drinks, remember to stock up on zero- or low-calorie drinks such as coffee, teas (this includes green tea), diet drinks, and water. Your zero- or no-calorie drinks, such as ginger tea, will give you a feeling of fullness during the fasting hours and help keep the hunger pangs at bay.

My advice to you is to remove all types of *temptation* within your eyesight, and what I mean by that is don't have chips and biscuits filling up your cupboard and have them be the first thing that you see when you open the cupboard. This is not to say that you should only eat *boring* food and remove all fun from your life. On IF, you can allow yourself a treat now and then, within reason, especially because, as you know, none of the plans stipulate exactly what foods to eat or avoid. The goal to keep in mind is to always make sure that you eat foods that provide optimum nutrition for your body and that you don't go over your weekly calorie allowance.

IF Side Effects

IF will have some side effects, so it will be very important to listen to your body for any clues and act accordingly. By this, I mean you must be patient with the process and take care of your body.

Listening to Your Body

Expect that your body may feel a bit different at the beginning as it adjusts to the new way of eating. You may experience symptoms such as nausea, vomiting, headaches, light-headedness, mental sluggishness, fatigue, and/or constipation. Generally, these side effects go away within a few days to a week of starting IF. It will be very important to listen to what your body is telling you and not ignore any danger signals. This is why throughout this book, I have been advising that you seek medical advice if you are not sure you are the right candidate for IF or if you experience any alarming symptoms. Definitely see a doctor if you experience abdominal pain, persistent nausea, and vomiting.

So what can you do to manage your symptoms and get through this challenging phase?

- *Stay hydrated*: Drink plenty of water. When your body goes into ketosis, your body gets rid of the water that was stored with the glycogen in the body cells, and when this happens, you will experience dehydration. This is why you need to rehydrate.
- *Electrolytes*: Your body loses electrolytes as it loses water. Many of these symptoms, such as headaches and fatigue, are a result of your body being low on electrolytes, and the easiest remedy for this is to add salt to your water or diet. Sea salt will be your best friend during this time. You can also hydrate with sports drinks that have electrolytes, but again, choose wisely and avoid those that are high in sugar.

- *Calories*: Not getting enough calories could be contributing to your symptoms, so make sure that you are getting enough to supply your daily needs. We discussed this in the above section, where we shared the tool for calculating your daily needs.
- *Supplements*: In relation to calories, it would also be beneficial to add supplements to your diet as your body may not be receiving enough nutrition as you cut down your calorie intake and stop eating certain foods. Consider a good multivitamin, as this will give your body the nutrients that it's not receiving from your diet.
- *Be gentle with yourself*: This is a transition period, so you have to take it easy and be gentle with yourself. This means avoiding strenuous activity for a while if you can. There are many gentler (low-impact) activities to choose from if you are a person who can't stay away from exercise, such as yoga. In Chapter 7, we go into detail on exercising while IF. Being gentle with yourself could also mean allowing yourself a small snack if your energy levels are dangerously low.

Making This Diet a Part of Your Lifestyle

In order for this to be a success, it is very important to take a look at your lifestyle and see how you are going to make IF work for you. Be honest with yourself. Are you the kind of person who eats out a lot? Do you have regular lunches with your coworkers, or do you have nights out with your friends and/or family? If so, then plan for your fasting window to coincide with these activities so that you can still partake in them instead of making excuses about why you can't go out with your friends anymore. Sometimes this could mean pushing your first meal of the day to be as late as possible in the day to allow yourself to have a late dinner. Having a pizza night? Save your calories by only having small snacks or one small meal during the day instead of a big meal. Plan in advance, and that way, you will feel that you have control over your diet instead of it controlling your life. If you fail to follow the guidelines once, don't beat yourself down and "throw the baby out with the bathwater." Make up for it in the following days. The goal is to enjoy yourself while you are on this diet and not to be miserable.

Chapter 7: Intermittent Fasting and Exercise

In the previous chapters, we briefly mentioned that combining IF with exercise is your best weapon in your battle to lose weight. In this chapter, we delve a little deeper into the mechanics of this.

What Are the Benefits of Exercise?

Combining ADF with exercise, specifically weight training, was shown to lead to significant decreases in weight, fat mass, waist circumference, and LDL (the bad cholesterol) while increasing HDL, the good cholesterol (Bhutani et al., 2013). Exercise also affects muscle biochemistry and metabolism, both of which are linked to insulin sensitivity and the management of blood sugar levels (Lindberg, 2020).

Autophagy Activation

A review of the literature shows that exercise seems to trigger autophagy (Jaspers et al., 2016). With autophagy, old cells are cleaned out to make way for newer and healthier cells to be produced by the body.

Antiaging Effects of Exercise

In relation to the above, cell regeneration has antiaging benefits, which means combining IF with exercise will give you the added benefit of longevity. We also mentioned earlier that IF boosts the production of HGH, so combining IF with exercise doubles its effects, and this enhances the production of collagen, which is great for your hair, nails, and joints.

When Is the Best Time to Exercise?

The experts seem to agree that working out first thing in the morning is the best time to exercise. Exercising on an empty stomach has the added advantage of going straight to your fat stores to start burning fat since, after a period of fasting, your glycogen stores will be almost depleted. This also supports your circadian rhythm (body clock), as working out late in the evening may disrupt your sleeping patterns. I recommend you don't eat immediately after exercise to optimize your hormone production. This recommendation is supported by some research that suggests that if you wait two to three hours after exercising to eat, this promotes the production of growth hormone, which, as we have discussed, also contributes to fat burning.

There are, however, some concerns that if you exercise on an empty stomach, your body might start breaking down proteins as fuel for energy, and you may not be able to *go hard* on your exercise as you will be low on energy. The timing of your exercise routine seems to be the key that unlocks the greatest benefits of exercise. Vieira et al. (2016) reviewed a number of key studies that compared the benefits of exercising in a fasted state versus a fed stomach, and they found that exercise performed in a fasted state led to higher fat oxidation.

What Type of Exercise Is Beneficial?

First, let's distinguish between the two types of exercise: *aerobic* vs. *anaerobic* exercise. Aerobic exercise is the type that increases your heart rate, but it is carried over a longer duration; think running, walking, etc. Anaerobic exercise, on the other hand, requires more effort but lasts for a short duration. A good example to think of here is lifting weights or sprinting.

Aerobic Exercise

Aerobic exercise, also referred to as cardio, can be done during fasting, but it's important to know that performance might drop a little, especially if you are new to exercising while doing IF. It could take up to six months to adapt one's endurance during IF. For this reason, it is not recommended for competing athletes to combine IF with training, especially just before a competing event, if it is their first time, as this may impact performance negatively.

High-Intensity Interval Training (HIIT)

This falls under the anaerobic category and has numerous benefits for the body, one of them being to promote the production of HGH. HIIT is also referred to as sprint training. Some of the benefits that HIIT provides the body with are "increased strength and stamina in the muscles and brain, increased growth hormone, improved body composition, increased brain function, higher testosterone levels, and less depression" (Prospect Medical, n.d.). Combining HIIT with IF will definitely give you the best results for weight loss and fat burning.

What About Weight Lifting?

Lifting weights definitely puts your body under a lot of stress, but doing it during your fasting window helps you burn through those glycogen stores and start burning fat. I suggest that you time your strength training closer to the end of your fasting window for this same reason and also because this will allow you to have a post-workout snack or meal soon after if you are the type who likes to have one. It's also very important to remember to stay hydrated during and after your workouts. Some people may also prefer to have a pre-workout snack, and even though this will *break* your fast, it may give you the energy boost that you need to maximize your training efforts. Just make sure that you don't choose from highly processed *energy bars* or *energy drinks,* as these are loaded with sugar, which would negate your weight loss efforts.

If you do a 24-hour fast, I recommend that you stick to low-intensity workouts simply because your energy levels will be super low. Think yoga, walking, Pilates, etc.

Most of the advice given here can be tailored to your personal preference. Everyone is different, and the important thing is to listen to your body and stop when you don't feel well or if you feel any type of pain in the middle of your training. Remember that it may take a couple of weeks for your body to adjust to training while doing IF, so you should go easy on yourself until you have found your own rhythm.

What to Eat During Exercise?

For pre and post-workout meals, I suggest you stick to wholesome foods. For your pre-workout snack, instead of reaching for an energy bar, you can have a slice of whole-grain toast and peanut or almond butter. The rule of thumb is to make sure that your meal consists of a complex carb and a protein, as in the example of toast and nut butter. For post-workout meals, you can include a carbohydrate, protein, and good fats, which this could be a chicken salad with olive oil.

What Are the Side Effects of Exercising While IF?

Exercising while fasting is not good for everyone, in the same way that IF isn't. Remember what we said earlier about stopping if you don't feel well. These are some of the negative effects that have been identified through research:

- According to a review done by the International Society of Sports Nutrition (ISSN), combining IF with exercise may lead to poorer performance, especially in athletes (Kerksick et al., 2017).
- Difficulties with building muscle: In an RCT, males who were put on IF for eight weeks while following a strength training program struggled to put on as much muscle as those who weren't doing IF (Tinsley et al., 2016). This doesn't mean that exercise will make you lose muscle, as a review of studies showed that IF helps with muscle maintenance (Varady, 2011).
- Combining IF with exercise may lead to a significant drop in sugar levels. IF alone contributes to low blood sugar levels due to the fewer meals, and so combining that with exercise may increase the impact, which could lead to fainting while performing an exercise.
- Almost related to the above point, some people may experience light-headedness while exercising, and this could also be triggered by low blood pressure as a result of combining exercise with IF.

The above are some of the things to bear in mind when you decide to include exercise in your diet regimen. Also, remember the special populations that we mentioned in earlier chapters that IF is not recommended for. We also do not recommend combining IF with exercise for that same group of people.

Chapter 8: Meal Planning

I n this chapter, I am going to share with you four types of meal plans: a beginner's plan, an intermediate plan, an advanced plan, and a 500-calorie day plan. This is to give you an example of what your daily meals could look like to help guide you in how to create your own plans. Remember that the plan you create must suit both your *health needs* and *lifestyle* for it to be a success, so always have that in mind as you create it.

Another tip I want to share with you is to see where you can use leftovers from your previous meals, as this helps cut down on the preparation time. If you cooked chicken a night or two before, use the leftovers to make a healthy salad for lunch the next day or a chicken sandwich. Be creative and have fun designing interesting meals. If you are unsure what the calorie count for your entire meal is and want to keep an eye on your calorie intake, here is another very handy and free tool I found at www.verywellfit.com/recipe-nutrition-analyzer-4157076.

With this tool, you can simply plug in the ingredients of your meal, and it will work out for you, not just the calories of the entire meal but the whole nutrient breakdown, including carbs, fats, and protein.

So let's look at some of the examples I have put together.

A Beginner's Meal Plan

As a newbie, you want to ensure that your meal plan is easy enough to follow without sabotaging your IF goals. What do I mean by that? Your meal plan should be easy enough to follow without overwhelming you with the planning involved. Secondly, you should not introduce many food products you are not familiar with because if you do that and realize later that you don't like them, this may discourage your efforts. Thirdly, it must not be so simple as to not look any different from the way you normally eat because, again, you may end up backsliding into your old ways of eating and end up back where you started. So my advice is to keep it simple, at least in the initial stages.

So here is one that I think would be suitable for beginners. We are going to base this plan on the Crescendo IF plan. Earlier in this book, we mentioned and listed the reasons why the Crescendo method is the best one for beginners. One of those reasons is that on this plan, you can start fasting anywhere from 12 to 16 hours. The following plan would be suitable for someone who is on a 10:14 plan.

Crescendo Plan for Beginners

Meal	Recipe	Ingredients	Directions
Breakfast or brunch (9–10 a.m.)	*Avocado Smoothie*	• 1/2 cup chopped avocado • 1 cup chopped spinach • ½ cup coconut milk • ½ cup milk • a handful of blueberries • 1 tbsp chia seeds • a handful of crushed ice	1. Blend everything in a high-speed blender. 2. Add ice cubes (optional). 3. Serve.
Lunch (1–2 p.m.)	*Avo–Ricotta Toast*	• ¼ cup ripe avocado, smashed • 1 slice whole-grain bread • 2 tbsp ricotta • salt and pepper to season • a pinch of crushed red pepper flakes	1. Toast bread. 2. Spread avocado and ricotta and sprinkle red pepper flakes, salt, and pepper on top. 3. Serve with scrambled egg or sliced boiled eggs on the side.
Dinner (6–7 p.m.)	*Spicy Salmon*	• 1½ lb wild Alaskan salmon, filleted • 4 medium tomatoes, diced • ½ cauliflower head (approx. 1 lb), cut into florets • 1 broccoli head (approx. 1 lb), cut into florets • taco seasoning • 3 tbsp oil • ½ tsp garlic powder	1. Preheat the oven to 375 °F. 2. Place the salmon in a baking dish. Mix the taco seasoning with ½ cup water in a small bowl and pour the mixture over the salmon. 3. Bake until opaque, should be 12–15 minutes. 4. In a food processor, pulse the cauliflower and broccoli until finely chopped and look like rice. 5. Heat the oil in a large skillet on medium heat and add the cauliflower and broccoli. Sprinkle with garlic powder, and cook for about 5–6 minutes until tender. 6. Serve the salmon with *rice* and garnish.

An Intermediate IF Plan

On this intermediate plan, you would have increased your fasting hours and decreased your *eating window*. So on the following proposed plan, you will eat from midday until 6 p.m. You may therefore have lunch as your first meal of the day, a healthy snack around midafternoon, and dinner at 6 p.m.

Meal	Recipe	Ingredients	Directions
Lunch (12 p.m.)	*Burgers*	• ½ lb ground beef liver • ½ lb ground beef • ½ tsp garlic powder • ½ tsp cumin powder • sea salt and pepper for seasoning • cooking oil for frying	1. Mix all the ingredients together in a bowl and form patties into desired size. 2. Heat cooking oil over the skillet on medium-high heat. 3. Fry burgers in a skillet until done. 4. Serve on a bed of greens and garnish. 5. Store extras in the refrigerator.
Snack (3 p.m.)	*Coconut Fat Bombs*	• ½ cup coconut cream • 2 tbsp almond butter • 1 tbsp coconut oil • 1 tsp cinnamon	1. Mix coconut cream with ½ tsp cinnamon. 2. Line an 8 x 8-inch square pan with parchment paper and spread coconut cream and cinnamon mixture at the bottom. 3. Combine ½ tsp cinnamon with coconut oil and almond butter. Spread this mixture over the first layer in the pan. 4. Put in the freezer for 10 minutes. Take out and cut into squares or bars as desired.
Dinner (6–7 p.m.)	*Chicken With Fried "Cauli" Rice*	• 1 ¼ lb chicken breast (boneless and skinless) • 2 tbsp grapeseed oil • 4 large eggs, whisked • 2 small carrots, finely chopped • 2 red bell peppers, finely chopped • 1 onion, finely chopped • 4 scallions, finely chopped • 2 cloves of garlic, finely chopped • ½ cup frozen peas (thawed) • 4 cups *cauli* rice • 2 tsp rice vinegar • 2 tbsp low-sodium soy sauce • salt and pepper to season	1. Heat 1 tbsp oil in a deep large skillet. Brown the chicken for about 3–4 minutes each side. Remove to cool off. 2. Add remaining oil in the skillet and scramble the eggs until set. Move to a bowl. 3. Add bell peppers, carrots, and onion onto the skillet and cook for approx. 5 minutes. Add the garlic and cook for another minute. Add the scallions and peas and toss together. 4. Add the cauliflower, rice vinegar, soy sauce, and seasoning. Combine well. 5. Allow the cauliflower to sit and brown without stirring for about 3 minutes. 6. Add the sliced chicken and egg.

An Advanced Meal Plan

The following plan is for those who have been doing IF for a while. These people may have advanced to the point where they are now practicing the 5:2 method, which means eating healthy meals for five days a week and observing complete 24-hour fasts for two days a week. So the following is an example of a plan you would use on your *non-fasting* days:

Meal	Recipe	Ingredients	Directions
Breakfast or brunch (10–11 a.m.)	*"Turkish" Eggs*	• 1 whole wheat pita • 5 large eggs • 2 tbsp yogurt • ¾ eggplant, diced • ¾ red bell pepper, diced • 2 tbsp olive oil • chopped cilantro • ¼ tsp paprika • salt and pepper to season	1. Heat the olive oil in a nonstick large pan. 2. Sauté the eggplant, bell pepper, salt, and pepper until soft, approx. 7 minutes. 3. Add eggs and paprika. Add more salt and pepper if needed. Cook till eggs are scrambled. 4. Sprinkle chopped cilantro and serve with a dollop of yogurt in the pita.
Snack (2–3 p.m.)	*Coconut Fat Bombs*	• ⅓ cup coconut oil • ⅔ cup smooth peanut butter • ½ cup dark cocoa • ½ cup coconut flakes, toasted • 4 packets sweetener (6 g) • 1 tbsp ground cinnamon • ¼ tsp kosher salt • ¼ tsp cayenne	1. In a boiler set over a pot of simmering water, mix coconut oil, peanut butter, and cocoa. Whisk until melted together and smooth. 2. Add sweetener, cinnamon, and salt, while stirring. 3. Spoon the mixture into mini muffin pans. 4. Sprinkle coconut and cayenne on top and put in the freezer for 30 minutes or until firm.
Dinner (6–7 p.m.)	*Oven-Baked Mahi-Mahi*	• 4 fillets of mahi-mahi • 1 cup mayonnaise • 1 lemon, juiced • ¼ cup white onion, finely chopped • ¼ tsp garlic salt • ¼ ground black pepper • breadcrumbs	1. Preheat the oven to 425 °F. 2. Clean the fish and place in a baking dish. 3. Squeeze lemon juice on the fish and sprinkle salt and pepper to taste. 4. On the side, mix mayonnaise with onion and spread on the fish. 5. Sprinkle the breadcrumbs on top and bake for approx. 25 minutes. 6. Serve with a salad of mixed greens or cauli rice.

A 500-Calorie Day Plan

If you are on the modified 5:2 plan or any of the other plans that are *modified*, so that instead of going for a complete 24-hour fast, you are allowed to eat no more than 500 calories on your fasting days, you may be wondering what that would look like. The following plan is an example of how you would schedule your meals and what they would look like on those days. We have provided you with four options for either a lunch or a snack to choose from, and if you combine any of those with the veggie dinner, it still keeps your calorie intake under 500 for the day.

Meal	Recipe	Ingredients	Directions
Lunch or snack (12 p.m.)	**Option 1:** *Berry Smoothie (323 calories)* **Option 2:** *Peach and Berry Smoothie (351.3 calories)* **Option 3:** *Baked Eggs With Veggies (114 calories)* **Option 4:** *Cauliflower "Popcorn" (156 calories)*	All recipes on Chapter 9	
Dinner (5 p.m.)	*Vegetable Curry (131 calories)*	• 1 onion, chopped • 1 lb butternut squash, peeled and cubed • 8 small cauliflowers, cut into florets • 2 parsnips, peeled and cubed • 2 oz French beans • 13 oz canned tomatoes, chopped • 16 oz vegetable stock • 3 tbsp Balti curry paste • 1 tbsp sunflower oil • salt and pepper to season	1. Heat the oil in a wok and add the onions. Fry for a few minutes until golden. Add the curry paste and stir for a few more minutes. 2. Add the butternut squash, parsnips, tomatoes, and vegetable stock. Boil and then lower the heat to simmer for about 10 minutes. 3. Add the cauliflower and cook for about 5 minutes then add the French beans. Cook for an additional 5 minutes until all vegetables are tender.

Now that I have presented you with some great meal plan examples, you have two options: You can either adopt any of my plans or just create using your own recipes or the ones provided in the next chapter. Have fun creating!

Chapter 9: Intermittent Fasting Recipes

I would like to think this is the chapter you have been dying to get to! I have literally taken the guesswork off of your *plate* by sourcing and providing some of the best recipes that are suitable for an IF life. Dig in and feel free to adjust to your needs and preferences.

Breakfast Recipes

Blueberry Compote Porridge

This is one of the easiest breakfast dishes you will ever make, and it will be ready in 10 minutes. It tastes really great and is very filling but low on calories. You have the option to either use fresh blueberries or frozen ones, which are cheaper and always handy to have in the freezer.

Time: 10 min

Serving size: 2

Prep time: 5 min

Cooking time: 5 min

Nutritional facts:

- Calories: 214
- Carbs: 35 g (7 g fiber)
- Fat: 4 g
- Protein: 13 g

Ingredients:

- 6 oz frozen blueberries
- 7 oz 0% fat natural yogurt
- 6 tbsp porridge oats
- 1 tsp honey (optional)

Directions:

1. Cook the oats with 14 oz water for about 2 minutes. Stir occasionally until thickened, and then remove from the heat. Add ⅓ of the yogurt.
2. In a separate pan, poach the blueberries until thawed using 1 tbsp of water and honey (if you are using it). Cook until tender but still holding shape.
3. Spoon the porridge into a serving bowl, top with the remaining yogurt, and spoon the blueberry compote on top.
4. Enjoy!

Scrambled Egg and Sweet Potatoes

This is a very tasty breakfast that you can use leftover vegetables from a previous meal to make, and it will take less than 30 minutes to prepare.

Time: 30 min

Serving size: 1

Prep time: 5 min

Cooking time: 25 min

Nutritional facts:

- Calories: 571
- Carbs: 52 g (9 g fiber)
- Fat: 20 g
- Protein: 44 g

Ingredients:

- 4 large eggs
- 4 large egg whites
- 1 (8 oz) sweet potato, cubed
- ½ cup onion, finely chopped
- 2 tsp chopped rosemary
- 2 tbsp chopped chives
- a shake of salt and pepper

Directions:

1. Preheat the oven to 425 °F (220 °C). Spray the baking sheet with cooking spray, and combine the sweet potato, onion, rosemary, and salt and pepper. Roast until tender, approximately 20 minutes.
2. Whisk the eggs, egg whites, and a pinch of salt and pepper in a mixing bowl. With cooking spray, spray the skillet and scramble the eggs on medium, for approximately 5 minutes.
3. Once done, add a sprinkle of chopped chives, and serve with the sweet potato mix.

Turmeric Tofu Scramble

This is a quick-and-easy recipe that is great for those times when you don't want to eat meat. Tofu is a great additional protein source.

Time: 15 min

Serving size: 1

Prep time: 5 min

Cooking time: 10 min

Nutritional facts:

- Calories: 431
- Carbs: 17 g
- Fat: 33 g
- Protein: 21 g

Ingredients:

- 1 portobello mushroom
- ½ avocado, thinly sliced
- ½ block (14 oz) firm tofu
- 3–4 pcs cherry tomatoes
- 1 tbsp olive oil and a little more for brushing
- ¼ tsp ground turmeric
- a pinch of garlic powder
- salt and pepper to season

Directions:

1. Preheat the oven to 400 °F (200 °C).
2. Place the mushroom and tomatoes on a baking sheet, and brush them with the olive oil. Season with salt and pepper, and roast until tender, approximately 10 minutes.
3. In a medium bowl, combine the tofu, ground turmeric, garlic powder, and a pinch of salt, and mash together with a fork.
4. Heat 1 tbsp olive oil in a large skillet over medium heat. Add the tofu mixture and cook. Stir occasionally until firm and it almost looks like an egg. This should take about 3 minutes.
5. Put the tofu on a plate, and serve with the mushroom, tomatoes, and avocado on the side.

Avocado Toast With Scrambled Egg

This is a delicious open-faced toast that packs the protein and the good fats from the avocado. This will have you eating in under 15 minutes.

Time: 15 min

Serving size: 1

Prep time: 10 min

Cooking time: 5 min

Nutritional facts:

- Calories: 501
- Carbs: 25.9 g
- Fat: 36.1 g
- Protein: 21.5 g

Ingredients:

- 2 eggs
- ½ avocado
- 1 slice sourdough bread, toasted
- 2 tbsp grated parmesan cheese (add more if preferred)
- 2 tbsp butter
- Dijon mustard

Directions:

1. Melt the butter in medium heat in a skillet and crack the eggs in. While the egg white is setting gently, break the egg yolks and scramble until completely cooked and firm. This should take about 3 minutes.
2. Spread Dijon mustard on one side of the sourdough bread.
3. Arrange avocado slices on the toast.
4. Gently place the cooked egg on top of the avocado.
5. Add a sprinkle of the parmesan cheese on top.
6. Serve.

Baked Eggs With Veggies

This recipe requires only three ingredients, is packed with protein, and will be ready in 20 minutes. You can start preparing it as you are about to finish your fast, and it will be ready in time for you to dig in.

Time: 20 min

Serving size: 4

Prep time: 5 min

Cooking time: 15 min

Nutritional facts:

- Calories: 114
- Carbs: 3 g
- Fat: 7 g
- Protein: 9 g

Ingredients:

- 4 eggs
- 14 oz (400 g) canned tomatoes, chopped
- 0.22 oz (100 g) bag of spinach
- 1 tsp chili flakes
- salt and pepper

Directions:

1. Heat oven to 300 °F (200 °C).
2. Wilt the leaves of the spinach by putting it in a colander and pouring over a kettle of boiling water. Squeeze out excess water, and divide the spinach into four small oven-proof dishes.
3. Combine the tomatoes, chili flakes, a bit of salt and pepper, and add to the spinach dishes. In the center of each dish, make a *well* and crack in an egg.
4. In the oven, bake for up to 15 minutes, depending on how you prefer your eggs.
5. Serve with warm toast (optional).

Berry Smoothie

A very filling smoothie that is nutrient dense and provides an alternative to the traditional *egg breakfast* option. This is ready in 5 minutes and is a great option for those who don't like to have bananas in their smoothies. Just a heads-up, this recipe requires a lot of ingredients so check that you have everything you need before you start.

Time: 5 min

Serving size: 1

Prep time: 5 min

Cooking time: NA

Nutritional facts:

- Calories: 323
- Carbs: 17.7 g
- Fat: 17.2 g
- Protein: 27.4 g

Ingredients:

- ¼ cup frozen or fresh blueberries
- ¼ cup frozen or fresh blackberries
- ¾ cup unsweetened almond milk
- ¼ cup fresh spinach
- 1 tsp coconut or MCT oil
- 1 tbsp chia seeds
- 2 tbsp Greek or coconut yogurt
- 1 scoop whey protein or collagen
- 1 tbsp unsweetened coconut (flaked) or flaked almonds
- 1 tsp cacao nibs
- 1 tsp flaxseed meal or hempseeds

Directions:

1. In a high-speed blender, whisk all the ingredients until smooth. Please note that using frozen berries and protein powder may make it a bit thick. In that case, just add more almond milk to make it thinner. Alternatively, use a mix of fresh and frozen berries.
2. Top with coconut flakes, flaxseed meal, blueberries, and cacao nibs.
3. Enjoy!

Lunch Recipes

Chicken Salad With Cheese

This is one of the quickest and easiest recipes to make, and you can use leftover chicken, if you had cooked it a night or two before. If you chill it the night before, you can save even more time.

Time: 35 min (including chill time)

Serving size: 1–2

Prep time: 35 min

Cooking time: NA

Nutritional facts:

- Calories: 364.5
- Carbs: 15.3 g
- Fat: 9.1 g
- Protein: 53.2 g

Ingredients:

- 1 cup cooked chicken breast (boneless and skinless), cubed
- ½ cup chopped baby spinach
- ¼ cup finely chopped celery
- ¼ cup carrot, shaved like ribbons
- 2 ½ tbsp nonfat mayonnaise
- 2 tbsp nonfat sour cream
- ⅛ tsp dried parsley
- 2 tsp Dijon mustard
- ¼ cup low-fat sharp cheddar cheese, shredded

Directions:

1. Mix the mayonnaise, sour cream, and Dijon mustard together.
2. Combine all ingredients in a bowl. Mix well and make sure all ingredients are well-coated with the mayonnaise mixture.
3. Chill in the fridge for about half an hour before you serve. Otherwise, chill the night before, and add the mayonnaise mix just before you serve.
4. Enjoy!

Chipotle Chicken "No"-wich

This on-the-go, *no-grain* lunchtime option takes 10 minutes to prepare and tastes great!

Time: 10 min

Serving size: 1

Prep time: 10 min

Cooking time: NA

Nutritional facts:

- Calories: 632
- Carbs: 12.7 g (6.1 g fiber)
- Fat: 48.5 g
- Protein: 38.3 g

Ingredients:

- 3 oz cooked chicken breast, shredded
- 2 tbsp mayonnaise
- 2 slices tomato
- 1 slice red onion
- ¼ avocado
- 1 tsp chipotle pepper in adobo sauce, minced
- 1 slice Havarti or cheddar cheese
- 6 lettuce leaves

Directions:

1. Mix the chicken with the mayonnaise and the chipotle pepper in a small bowl.
2. Put a piece of parchment paper on the table and lay the lettuce leaves, slightly overlapping each other. Top the lettuce with the chicken–mayonnaise mix. Top with the remaining ingredients.
3. Roll the wrap using the lettuce leaves.
4. Roll tightly and cut in half. Eat immediately, or secure with tape, if you are taking it away for a later lunch.

Cajun Potato and Prawn Salad

Delicious prawn or shrimp dish for seafood lovers, this one is very easy and quick to prepare.

Time: 30 min

Serving size: 2

Prep time: 10 min

Cooking time: 20 min

Nutritional facts:

- Calories: 435.6
- Carbs: 37.9 g (fiber 10.8 g)
- Fat: 23 g
- Protein: 23.1 g

Ingredients:

- 10 oz new potatoes, halved
- 8 oz king prawns, peeled and cooked
- 2 spring onions, finely sliced
- 1 clove garlic, minced
- 1 avocado, diced
- 1 tbsp olive oil
- 2 tsp Cajun seasoning
- a cup of alfalfa sprout
- salt (for boiling potatoes)

Directions:

1. Cook the potatoes in lightly salted boiling water for approximately 10 minutes until tender. Drain.
2. Heat the olive oil in a skillet and add prawns, spring onions, and Cajun seasoning. Stir-fry until the prawns are hot, for about 2 minutes.
3. Add in the potatoes, and cook for another minute.
4. Spoon onto serving dish, and garnish with avocado and the alfalfa sprouts.
5. Serve.

Lunch Wraps

These wraps can be made in a batch and frozen, so when you are going to the office, you would just grab one or two on your way out. They can be easily enjoyed with family too.

Time: 1 hr 5 min

Serving size: 16 wraps

Prep time: 30 min

Cooking time: 35 min

Nutritional facts:

- Calories: 557
- Carbs: 80.8 g (4.2 g fiber)
- Fat: 16 g
- Protein: 22.9 g

Ingredients:

- 4 cups water
- 2 cups brown rice (uncooked)
- 16 (10 in) flour tortillas
- 1 lb pepper Jack cheese, shredded
- 4 cans (15 oz) black beans
- 2 cans (15.5 oz) pinto beans
- 1 can (10 oz) whole kernel corn
- 1 can (10 oz) diced tomatoes and green chilies

Directions:

1. In a saucepan, combine the water and rice and bring to a boil. Reduce to low heat, cover, and simmer for 35–40 minutes. Put aside to cool.
2. Strain the black beans and the pinto beans in a colander and rinse. Toss with the tomato and green chilies and corn to mix. Transfer to a larger bowl, and add the rice and cheese.
3. Divide evenly onto the tortillas, and roll up tightly. Wrap individually in plastic and freeze in a bag what you don't need right away.
4. Reheat in the microwave on the day you want to eat.

Cabbage Meat "Cutlets"

The best thing about these *cutlets* is that not only are they tasty, but you can make them in a batch and freeze for use later. You can also serve them with grilled veggies or a side salad.

Time: 50 min

Serving size: 6

Prep time: 10 min

Cooking time: 40 min

Nutritional facts:

- Calories: 449
- Carbs: 6.3 g
- Fat: 35 g
- Protein: 26.2 g

Ingredients:

- ½ medium cabbage (hard core removed) or kale
- 1 small red onion
- 1.1 lb ground beef
- 2 large eggs
- 2 tbsp lard
- 2 cloves garlic
- ½ Himalayan salt
- freshly ground pepper
- 2 tsp marjoram
- fresh parsley (for garnish)
- lemon wedges (for garnish)

Directions:

1. Preheat the oven to 400 °F.
2. Boil a large pot of water with salt. Cut the cabbage into quarters, and place in the boiling water. Cook for 12–15 minutes.
3. Peel and dice the onion and garlic. Heat the lard and fry them for 3–4 minutes until golden.
4. In a separate bowl, add the mince and eggs. Season with salt and pepper, marjoram, and the onion and garlic mix. Combine well.
5. When the cabbage is soft, put aside to cool down. Drain well using a kitchen towel to remove excess water. Remove any hard pieces, and chop into small pieces.
6. Add the cabbage into the mince mixture using your hands to combine well. Divide into small, palm-sized *cutlets*.
7. Place the cutlets on an ovenproof baking dish using a bit of lard to grease it first.
8. Bake for about 20–25 minutes.
9. Serve with lemon wedges and fresh parsley and sour cream (optional). Alternatively, serve with a small side salad.
10. The cutlets can be stored in the fridge for up to four days or frozen for up to three months.

Chickpea Curry

This recipe is great for when you don't want to eat meat, and it's packed with protein-rich ingredients. It's also great for winter lunches or dinners.

Time: 55 min

Serving size: 6

Prep time: 15 min

Cooking time: 40 min

Nutritional facts:

- Calories: 204
- Carbs: 20 g
- Fat: 7 g
- Protein: 11 g

Ingredients:

- 1 (400 g/14 oz) can drained chickpeas
- 6 ripe tomatoes
- 1 (100 g or 0.22 oz) bag baby spinach leaves
- 1 onion, chopped
- 1 in piece grated ginger
- 2 garlic cloves, chopped
- ½ tbsp olive oil
- 1 tsp ground cumin
- 2 tsp ground coriander

- 1 tsp turmeric
- 1 pinch chili flakes
- 1 tsp yeast extract (can use Marmite)
- 4 tbsp red lentils
- 6 tbsp coconut cream
- 1 head of broccoli, broken into small florets
- 1 lemon, cut into half
- 1 tbsp toasted sesame seeds
- 1 tbsp cashews, chopped (mix it with the sesame seeds)

Directions:

1. Blend the onion, garlic, ginger, and tomatoes in a food processor or blender to a nice thick purée.
2. In a large pan, heat oil, add the spices, and fry for a few seconds. Add the purée and yeast extract. Allow the mixture to bubble for about 2 minutes.
3. Add the lentils and coconut cream, and cook until the lentils are soft. Add the broccoli and cook for another 4–5 minutes.
4. Stir in the drained chickpeas and spinach, add a squeeze of lemon, and add in the sesame and cashew mixture.
5. Serve with brown rice (optional).

Dinner Recipes

Quick Leftover Stir-Fry

This stir-fry is quick and easy to make during the week, especially if you are making dinner for one. The meat and the vegetables can all be leftovers from a previous meal which will shorten preparation time.

Time: 25 min

Serving size: 1

Prep time: 10 min

Cooking time: 15 min

Nutritional facts:

- Calories: 480
- Carbs: 74.9 g (4.2 g fiber)
- Fat: 11 g
- Protein: 19.5 g

Ingredients:

- 1 chicken breast
- ½–1 cup cooked leftover rice (brown rice)
- 1 cup frozen stir-fry vegetables (any variant)
- 1–2 tbsp olive oil
- spices for seasoning (optional)
- a pinch of Himalayan salt and pepper

Directions:

1. Cut the chicken breast into strips. Spice it with your favorite meat spices, salt, and pepper (if not already cooked).
2. Fry in olive oil until golden.
3. Add stir-fry vegetables, and toss together for another 5–10 minutes.
4. Add cooked rice and combine well. Season to taste.
5. Serve.

Easy Baked Cod

This baked cod is easy and quick to make and can be enjoyed by the whole family. Can be served with a side of veggies or salad. Otherwise, eat half of it, and keep it in the fridge for the next day's lunch.

Time: 30 min

Serving size: 4

Prep time: 10 min

Cooking time: 20 min

Nutritional facts:

- Calories: 236
- Carbs: 13 g (1 g fiber)
- Fat: 6 g
- Protein: 30 g

Ingredients:

- 4 cod loin fillets
- 3 tbsp flour
- 2 tbsp olive oil
- 1 lemon, sliced
- ½ small bunch of thyme
- salt and pepper to season

Directions:

1. Preheat the oven to 430 °F.
2. In a bowl, mix the flour with seasoning, and coat each side of the cod fillets.
3. In a nonstick pan, heat the oil, and fry the cod on each side for about 2 minutes or until golden brown.
4. Transfer the fillets into a roasting pan. Arrange the lemon slices, and sprinkle the thyme on top of the fish. Drizzle with remaining oil, and bake for about 10 minutes.
5. Once done, serve with a side of grilled veggies or a salad.

Spaghetti Bolognese

This recipe can be made as a vegetarian option by substituting ground turkey with soya meat.

Time: 1 hr 30 min

Serving size: 4

Prep time: 1 hr

Cooking time: 30 min

Nutritional facts:

- Calories: 450
- Carbs: 31 g (6 g fiber)
- Fat: 23 g
- Protein: 32 g

Ingredients:

- 1¼ lb ground turkey
- 1 large spaghetti squash
- 1 (8 oz) can low-sodium, sugar-free tomato sauce
- 3 cups fresh tomatoes, chopped (or 2 15-oz cans)
- 1 small onion, finely chopped
- 3 tbsp olive oil
- ½ tsp garlic powder
- kosher or Himalayan salt and pepper
- 4 cloves garlic, chopped
- basil, freshly chopped

Directions:

1. Preheat the oven to 400 °F.
2. While the oven is heating, cut the spaghetti squash in half lengthwise, and throw away the seeds. Rub each half with 1/2 tbsp oil, garlic powder, and ¼ tsp each of salt and pepper. Place with the skin-side up on a rimmed baking sheet, and roast until soft, approximately 35–40 minutes. Allow to cool for 10 minutes.
3. In a large skillet, heat the remaining 2 tbsp oil on medium heat. Add the onion and season with ¼ tsp each of salt and pepper. Cook, stirring occasionally, until soft, for about 6 minutes. Add the turkey in and cook, while breaking it up into small pieces with a spoon until browned. This should take about 6–7 minutes. Add the garlic and cook for 1 minute.
4. Move the turkey mixture to one side of the pan, and add the mushrooms on to the other half. Cook the mushrooms until tender, stirring occasionally, for about 5 minutes, and then mix with the turkey. Now, add the tomatoes and tomato sauce, and simmer for another 10 minutes.
5. Scoop out the squash, and transfer onto the plates while the sauce is simmering. Spoon the turkey Bolognese over the top, and sprinkle with basil, if so desired.

Carrot and Lentil Soup

This recipe would be a great choice for those who are vegetarian, and it is easy to prepare. It would be great for winter nights too.

Time: 25 min including prep time

Serving size: 4

Prep time: 10 min

Cooking time: 15 min

Nutritional facts:

- Calories: 238
- Carbs: 34
- Fat: 7 g
- Protein: 11 g

Ingredients:

- 21 oz coarsely grated carrots, washed and unpeeled
- 5 oz split red lentils
- 33 oz hot vegetable stock
- 4 oz milk (or a nondairy variant)
- 2 tbsp olive oil
- plain yogurt and naan bread, for serving
- 2 tsp cumin seeds
- a pinch of chili flakes

Directions:

1. In a large saucepan, dry fry the cumin seeds and chili flakes for about 1 minute, until they release their aromas.
2. Set aside about half of it. Add the olive oil, grated carrots, red lentils, vegetable stock, and milk to the pan, and bring to the boil.
3. Let it simmer for about 15 minutes until the lentils are swollen and softened.
4. Using a blender, whisk the soup ingredients until smooth, or pour into a food processor and blend to the desired consistency.
5. Season to your preferred taste, and add a dollop of the plain yogurt. Add a sprinkling of the toasted spices you reserved earlier. Enjoy with warmed naan bread.

Baked Chicken and Brussels Sprouts

This delicious, easy chicken dinner is suitable for one, to eat over two meals or more, or for a small family. This one is also very low on calories.

Time: 40 min

Serving size: 4

Prep time: 15 min

Cooking time: 25 min

Nutritional facts:

- Calories: 323.4
- Carbs: 7.9 g (2.5 g fiber)
- Fat: 24.8 g
- Protein: 17.6 g

Ingredients:

- 4 chicken thighs (with skin on)
- 4 carrots, cut on a bias
- 1 ½ cups brussels sprouts, halved
- 3 tbsp olive oil
- 1 tsp herbes de Provence
- salt and pepper to season

Directions:

1. Heat oven to 400 ºF.
2. In a bowl, mix the already cut vegetables with ½ tsp herbs, 1 ½ tbsp olive oil, and seasoning. Make sure the veggies are well coated.
3. Place vegetables in a sheet pan.
4. Now, place the chicken in the bowl, and add the remaining herbs and olive oil, and rub the chicken well.
5. Place the chicken onto the sheet pan.
6. Roast for 30–35 minutes, until the chicken is done.
7. If you like your chicken browner, put the oven to broil for about 2 minutes.
8. Take out and serve.

Grilled Salmon

This meal is suitable for either lunch or dinner. It takes a bit of time to prepare as it requires chilling time. It would be best to prepare when you are not in a hurry, maybe on the weekends.

Time: 1 hr 20 min

Serving size: 4

Prep time: 1 hr

Cooking time: 20 min

Nutritional facts:

- Calories: 380.7
- Carbs: 17.3 g
- Fat: 17.9 g
- Protein: 37 g

Ingredients:

- 1 1/2 lb salmon fillets
- 1/4 cup packed brown sugar
- 1 chicken bouillon cube mixed with 3 tbsp water
- 3 tbsp olive oil (or any preferred)
- 3 tbsp soy sauce
- 4 tbsp green onions, finely chopped
- 1 lemon, thinly sliced
- 2 slices onion, separated into rings
- 2 tsp fresh dill
- 1/2 tsp each of salt and pepper
- 1/2 tsp garlic powder

Directions:

1. Season salmon fillets with dill, pepper, salt, and garlic powder.
2. Spray with nonstick spray, and place in a shallow glass pan.
3. Combine sugar, chicken bouillon, oil, soy sauce, and green onions, and pour over salmon.
4. Cover and chill for 1 hour, turning once.
5. Drain the marinade.
6. Grill on medium heat, and place lemon and onion on top.
7. Cover and cook for a further 15 minutes or until the fish is well done.
8. Serve with a side of roast veggies or salad.

Healthy Snacks

Almond and Apple Muffins

If you love muffins, this is a great way to enjoy them as a healthy snack, not the store-bought types that are laden with sugar. Make these in a batch, and keep them in the refrigerator for when you need to grab a quick bite.

Time: 20 min

Serving size: 5

Prep time: 8 min

Cooking time: 12 min

Nutritional facts:

- Calories: 484
- Carbs: 16 g (5 g fiber)
- Fat: 31 g
- Protein: 40 g

Ingredients:

- 2 cups almond meal
- 4 large eggs
- 4 scoops vanilla protein powder
- ½ stick butter
- 1 cup unsweetened applesauce
- 2 tsp baking powder
- 1 tbsp cinnamon
- 1 tsp allspice
- 1 tsp cloves

Directions:

1. Preheat the oven to 350 °F.
2. Put the butter in a small microwave bowl, and melt it in the microwave for approximately 30 seconds on low heat.
3. Combine all the remaining ingredients with the melted butter in a large bowl. Mix thoroughly.
4. Using nonstick cooking spray, spray two muffin pans or use cupcake liners, if you have them.
5. Pour the dough into the muffin pans. Be careful not to overfill them (three fourths full should be fine as they will rise). The dough should be enough to make 10 muffins.
6. Place and bake one tray at a time in the oven. Bake each for about 12 minutes. Make sure not to over bake the muffins; they will become too dry if you do.
7. Enjoy as a snack with butter, and store in the refrigerator.

Peach and Berry Smoothie

We all love a good smoothie, especially during the summer months. Here is a very simple but delicious and healthy smoothie that takes less than 10 minutes to make. You can also have this as your post-workout *meal*.

Time: 5 min

Serving size: 1

Prep time: 5 min

Cooking time: NA

Nutritional facts:

- Calories: 351.3
- Carbs: 61.6 g (4.5 g fiber)
- Fat: 12.4 g
- Protein: 2.7 g

Ingredients:

- a cup of frozen peaches
- 1/2 cup Greek yogurt
- 1/4 cup coconut milk (depending on how thick or thin you like it)
- 1/2 tsp almond flavoring

Directions:

1. Mix everything in a blender at high speed.
2. Check the thickness, and adjust as per your preference. You should add more milk if you want it thinner and more peaches if you want the smoothie thicker.
3. Top with chia seeds, berries, and almonds.

Cauliflower "Popcorn"

This very healthy snack feels like an indulgence but is full of goodness and easy to make. You need a bit of planning time for this because it takes a while in the oven, so don't make it when you're famished.

Time: 1 hr 10 min

Serving size: 4

Prep time: 10 min

Cooking time: 1 hr

Nutritional facts:

- Calories: 156
- Carbs: 7.3 g (2.9 g fiber)
- Fat: 13.9 g
- Protein: 2.8 g

Ingredients:

- 1 head cauliflower or an equal amount of commercially prepared cauliflower
- 4 tbsp olive oil
- salt to season

Directions:

1. Preheat the oven to 425 °F.
2. Prepare the head of the cauliflower, remove the core and the thick stems, and cut the florets into small pieces (each one the size of a small ball).
3. Combine the olive oil and salt in a large bowl, whisk together, and add the cauliflower pieces in. Toss thoroughly.
4. Line a baking sheet with parchment paper, and spread the cauliflower pieces on the sheet. Roast for 1 hour, turning a few times until the pieces have turned golden brown. The browner or golden they are, the sweeter the taste.
5. Serve in a bowl, and enjoy it like *popcorn*.

Broccoli Crunchies

Got broccoli in the fridge? Make this delicious healthy snack that takes just 10 minutes to prepare. This recipe is enough for four servings which means you can reserve some in the fridge, so when you have the munchies again, instead of reaching out for a packet of crisps, you can have this.

Time: 22 min

Serving size: 4

Prep time: 7 min

Cooking time: 15 min

Nutritional facts:

- Calories: 172.7
- Carbs: 7 g (0.2 g fiber)
- Fat: 15.8 g
- Protein: 4.1 g

Ingredients:

- 1 lb broccoli
- 2 tbsp unsalted butter
- 1–2 tbsp lemon juice
- 2 tbsp olive oil
- 1 tsp garlic, minced
- ½ tsp lemon zest
- 2 tbsp pine nuts, toasted
- salt and ground pepper (to season)

Directions:

1. Preheat the oven to 500 °F.
2. Toss the broccoli florets in a bowl with olive oil and the salt and pepper for seasoning.
3. On a baking sheet, arrange the broccoli florets in a single layer. Turn once. Roast for about 12 minutes or until tender.
4. While you wait for the broccoli to get ready, melt the butter in a small pot over medium heat.
5. Add the garlic and lemon zest to the butter while heating, and stir for about a minute.
6. Cool off slightly then add the lemon juice to the mixture.
7. Spoon the broccoli into a serving dish, drizzle with the garlic–lemon, and toss together until well coated.
8. Sprinkle the toasted pine nuts on top and serve.

Sweet or Savory Waffles

These waffles can be enjoyed as a delicious sweet treat or savory, depending on what you fancy. The ingredients can also be substituted according to what you have, such as using butter instead of coconut oil. They are low in carbs and are ready in 10 minutes. Make a batch and keep in the fridge for later use. This can be stored for up to five days in the fridge.

Time: 15 min

Serving size: 2

Prep time: 10 min

Cooking time: 5 min

Nutritional facts:

- Calories: 299
- Carbs: 5.6 g (2.9 g fiber)
- Fat: 21.2 g
- Protein: 19 g

Ingredients:

- ¼ coconut flour
- 2 large eggs
- ½ almond milk
- 1 scoop (¼ cup) whey protein or egg white protein powder
- ¼ tsp baking soda
- 2 tbsp butter or coconut oil or ghee
- ½ tsp apple cider vinegar or cream of tartar
- a pinch of pink Himalayan salt

Directions:

1. Add all the dry ingredients into a mixing bowl, and mix them well. You may need to sift the coconut flour.
2. In a separate bowl, crack the eggs and mix with almond milk and melted coconut oil, and whisk together well.
3. Add the dry ingredients into the egg mixture, and combine well.
4. Spoon the batter into the waffle maker, and cook for about 2 minutes.
5. Once done, place on your serving plate.
6. Top off with ingredients of your choice.

Mocha Pots

Have a sweet tooth? Here is a very easy to make and delicious snack or dessert that takes less than 10 minutes to make.

Just a heads-up, this snack is not very low on calories, so eat this on the days you are watching your calorie intake, so you won't overdo it. I would recommend having this no more than once or twice a month as a treat.

Time: 10 min

Serving size: 4

Prep time: 5 min

Cooking time: 2 min

Nutritional facts:

- Calories: 676
- Carbs: 28 g (1 g fiber)
- Fat: 60 g
- Protein: 5 g

Ingredients:

- 7 oz milk or dark chocolate with coffee (broken into chunks)
- 10 oz double cream
- 2 tbsp creme fraiche
- 1 tsp vanilla extract

Directions:

1. In a microwave, melt the chocolate for about 2 minutes. Alternatively, do this on the stovetop over a pan of simmering water. Leave aside to cool off for a bit.
2. Whip the double cream with the vanilla extract in a separate bowl until lightly whipped. Now fold in the melted, cooled chocolate until well combined.
3. Spoon the mixture into four small bowls or ramekins, and serve with a dollop of creme fraiche on top.
4. If you will be serving later, just keep in the fridge, and add the creme fraiche when it's serving time. Enjoy!

Vegetarian Recipes

Broccoli and Dhal Curry

This beautiful vegetarian curry is packed with flavor and may be more suitable for winter nights or lunches. It is low on calories and packed with protein.

Time: 1 hr 30 min

Serving size: 4

Prep time: 30 min

Cooking time: 1 hr

Nutritional facts:

- Calories: 445
- Carbs: 59 g (15.1 g fiber)
- Fat: 15.4 g
- Protein: 25.7 g

Ingredients:

- 2 medium-sized onions
- 4 tbsp butter or ghee
- 1 cup red lentils
- 2 medium broccoli, chopped
- 3 cups of chicken broth
- 1 lemon, juiced
- 1 tbsp flour

- ½ cup ground coconut (optional)
- 2 tsp cumin
- 2 tsp turmeric
- 1 tsp ground coriander
- 1 tsp chili powder
- 1 ½ tsp ground black pepper
- 1 tsp salt
- 1 cup coarsely chopped cashews (optional)

Directions:

1. Heat the butter and sauté the onions until golden.
2. Add the spices (turmeric, cumin, coriander, pepper, and chili powder) and cook, stirring for about a minute.
3. Add lemon juice, lentils, broth, and coconut (if using).
4. Bring the pot to boil, reduce the heat, and simmer for about 55 minutes. Add water if too thick.
5. In a separate pan, steam broccoli for approximately 7 minutes. Dip in cold water and set aside.
6. Remove a ⅓ cup amount from the lentil soup, and make a paste using the flour.
7. Return to the pan, and add salt, broccoli, and nuts, if using them.
8. Simmer for another 5 minutes.
9. Serve with cauli rice or basmati rice.

Green Soup

A low-calorie soup that is packed with nutrient-dense vegetables as a nice lunchtime option.

Time: 35 min

Serving size: 2

Prep time: 15 min

Cooking time: 20 min

Nutritional facts:

- Calories: 182
- Carbs: 14 g (5 g fiber)
- Fat: 8 g
- Protein: 10 g

Ingredients:

- 2 cups of stock (make with bouillon and boiling water)
- ½ lb (200 g) zucchini, roughly sliced
- 3 oz (85 g) broccoli
- 3.5 oz (100 g) kale, chopped
- 1 tbsp oil
- 1 lime (zest and juice)
- 2 small cloves garlic, sliced
- 1 piece of ginger (thumb size)
- ½ tsp ground coriander
- ½ tsp ground turmeric
- a pinch of Himalayan salt
- a small pack of parsley, chopped roughly

Directions:

1. In a deep pan using the oil, fry the garlic, ginger, coriander, turmeric, and salt on medium heat for 2 minutes. Add 3 tablespoons of water to add a bit of moisture.
2. Add the zucchini, and mix well with the spices, and fry for about 3 minutes. Add approximately ⅖ of the stock, and let it simmer for about 3 minutes.
3. Add the kale, broccoli, and lime juice with the rest of the stock, and let it simmer for a further 3 minutes until soft.
4. Remove from the heat, and add the chopped parsley. Pour into a blender, and blend on high speed until smooth and to the desired thickness.
5. Serve garnished with lime zest and bits of parsley.

Easy Pizza

Who said you can't eat pizza on the IF diet? Now for a guilt-free indulgence, you can get your hands dirty and make your own pizza at home. This pizza crust is almost carb-free, and you can top it with your favorite toppings! Get creative, but please remember that the nutritional info provided for this recipe is for the crust only, so be careful with your toppings.

Time: 1 hr 10 min

Serving size: 4

Prep time: 20 min

Cooking time: 50 min

Nutritional facts:

- Calories: 45.3
- Carbs: 5.6 g (2.2 g fiber)
- Fat: 1.5 g
- Protein: 3.6 g

Ingredients:

- 4 cups of raw cauliflower (riced) or 1 medium head
- 1 cup chèvre or soft cheese
- 1 egg, beaten
- 1 tsp oregano
- 1 pinch salt

Directions:

1. Preheat the oven to 400 °F.
2. Make the *cauli* rice in a food processor by breaking down the florets, if not using the ready-mix packet.
3. Boil an inch of water in a pot, add the *rice,* and cook for about 4 minutes, then drain.
4. Transfer to a dish towel and squeeze out the extra water. This is to make sure the crust comes out nice and dry (also stable).
5. Mix the *rice*, egg, cheese, and spices. Mix the dough well with your hands.
6. Line a baking sheet with parchment paper, and lay out the dough nicely into a round shape. Try to keep it about ⅜ in thickness.
7. Bake for approximately 35–40 minutes, until firm and golden brown.
8. Take it out, and add your favorite toppings: different cheeses, veggies, etc.
9. Return to the oven for up to 10 minutes, until the cheese is bubbling.
10. Slice and serve with a side salad (optional).

"Spanish" Omelet or Tortilla

This version of the *Spanish omelette* can be served as a tortilla for a great, tasty lunch option that's packed with flavor.

Time: 45 min

Serving size: 4

Prep time: 20 min

Cooking time: 25 min

Nutritional facts:

- Calories: 241
- Carbs: 11 g
- Fat: 17 g
- Protein: 11 g

Ingredients:

- ½ lb new potatoes, thickly sliced with ends trimmed
- 1 small onion, halved and sliced
- 6 large eggs
- 3 tbsp olive oil
- 2 cloves garlic, chopped
- ½ tsp smoked paprika
- 3 tbsp parsley, chopped, or ½ tsp dried oregano
- salt and pepper to season

Directions:

1. In a deep pan, heat the oil and fry the onion, potatoes, and garlic for about 10 minutes. Add paprika and fry for another minute.
2. Whisk the eggs with the dried or fresh herbs, and add seasoning. Pour into the pan.
3. Stir a few times, and let the egg set at the bottom. Leave to cook on very low heat for about 10 minutes until set, except the top part.
4. Transfer the *tortilla* onto the plate, and carefully lift and turn back into the saucepan so that the part that was at the bottom is now on top. You are now cooking the top part. Cook for about 2 minutes.
5. Transfer to a plate, garnish with parsley, and serve, or alternatively wrap in foil and serve warm like a tortilla.

Quinoa and Veggie Lunch

This quinoa and veggie lunch is easy to make and will be ready to eat in 30 minutes. It's a great option when preparing a meal for one. It's also very low on calories.

Time: 30 min

Serving size: 1

Prep time: 10 min

Cooking time: 20 min

Nutritional facts:

- Calories: 225
- Carbs: 41.1 g
- Fat: 3.3 g
- Protein: 10.2 g

Ingredients:

- ¼ cup red quinoa (or white if preferred)
- ½ cup water
- ½ cup carrots, thinly sliced
- 1 cup cooked broccoli, chopped
- 1 cup baby spinach, chopped
- ½ tsp chicken bouillon granules

Directions:

1. Add water, carrots, quinoa, and bouillon to a decent-sized saucepan, and cook over medium heat. When it starts boiling, reduce the heat, and let it simmer until all the water is absorbed. The outer ring of the quinoa grain must be visible. This should take about 12 minutes.
2. Add spinach and broccoli, and close the pot. Let the spinach wilt. Cook until all the water has been absorbed and all the veggies are heated through. This should take about 5 minutes.
3. Spoon the quinoa mix into a bowl and serve.

Vegetarian Chili

This vegetarian chili is so easy to make, and you have the option to skip the meat substitute and just use the beans only, and it will still taste great. You can also reduce the number of onions to your preference. This is great for winter nights. Since it is enough for six, you can freeze and use again at a later stage.

Time: 1 hr 10 min

Serving size: 6

Prep time: 10 min

Cooking time: 1 hr

Nutritional facts:

- Calories: 582
- Carbs: 74.2 g
- Fat: 4.9 g
- Protein: 67.5 g

Ingredients:

- 2 cans (15 oz) black beans
- 2 cans (15 oz) dark red kidney beans
- 1 can (15 oz) light red kidney beans
- 1 can (29 oz) diced tomatoes
- 1 can (12 fl oz) tomato juice
- 1 package (12 oz) frozen burger-style crumbles
- 5 onions (reduce if preferred)
- 3 tbsp chili powder
- 1 tbsp garlic powder
- 1 ½ tbsp ground cumin
- 2 bay leaves
- salt and pepper to season

Directions:

1. Combine all the ingredients into one large pot, and allow to simmer. Cover and cook for about an hour.
2. Serve.

Chapter 10: Debunking Some of the Common Intermittent Fasting Myths

In this chapter, we are going to discuss some of the myths surrounding IF, as I am certain that you may have heard most of them. From personal experience, most myths are usually started by uninformed people who have not done their research or have not tried the diet themselves, who spread the stories that they have heard through other people. Some myths are based on anecdotes and not actual science. One person knows someone who had a bad experience, and that is turned into a *fact* about the diet. My hope is that this chapter will help *put those to bed* by sharing facts in the place of myths.

On IF, You Can Eat Whatever You Like

You have probably heard this one as it is the most popular one, and that's why I'm starting with it. As you will know by now, throughout this book, I have been emphasizing the importance of choosing foods that are packed with nutrients that feed your body and making sure that you stay within your calorie allowance so as not to negate the effects of IF. If you eat whatever you like and binge during your eating window, this will be counterproductive to what you are trying to achieve. That is why in Chapter 6, we spoke about the importance of defining and stating your reason for doing this diet right at the beginning, as this will help you stay the course. We also shared some tips for the times when you want to treat yourself to a pizza night with friends. This diet is meant to help you adopt good eating habits, not to encourage irresponsible eating behavior, which may lead to eating disorders.

All IF Is the Same

If all IF were the same, we wouldn't have a whole chapter dedicated to the different types and IF plans. Very early in this book, we discussed the three categories: ADF, TRF, and periodic fasting, as well as the different plans that fall under each one. As much as they all share common health benefits in terms of fat burning, insulin regulation, brain health, etc., we also discussed the specific benefits that each one offers. Most uninformed people think IF means just skipping a meal, such as those who believe that all you have to do is just skip breakfast, and you can call yourself someone who practices IF. At this point, you know that none of that is true, and next time someone says this, you can kindly correct that misconception.

You Cannot Exercise While You Are IF

This, as we know, is not true. In this book, we have discussed extensively the numerous studies that have shown the benefits of combining IF with exercise. We also discussed the added benefit of exercising on an empty stomach, which is to burn the fat stores, as the glycogen stores are usually at their lowest by that time. This myth, we suspect, comes from the belief that you will be very low on energy and therefore unable to exercise, but again, we discussed the measures that you can take to counter this, such as having a pre-workout or a post-workout snack soon after your training. Or you can schedule your breakfast soon after your training.

IF Slows Down Your Metabolism

This comes from the school of thought that says frequently eating during the day cranks up your metabolism, causing your body to burn fat. This is based on the often misunderstood thermic effect of food (TEF) which is the calories your body expends to process the food you ingest. What is misunderstood though, is that TEF is only 10% of what you consume, and this is not enough to burn a significant amount of fat.

The myth that IF slows down your metabolism has been proven untrue by different studies looking into this (Moro et al., 2016). People who spread this myth do not understand that IF is not about restricting calories, but rather, it's about restricting the number of hours you are taking food in. A decrease in metabolism would be triggered by a severe limitation of calorie intake, and that happens when you are undereating. IF is not about undereating but rather eating at certain scheduled periods to allow your body some downtime to process the food.

IF Only Works Because Your Body Doesn't Process Food

People who say this obviously don't know that even when there is *no food* for your body to process at night or while you are fasting, your body is still working because other bodily processes are running in the background. In the early chapters, we discussed one of these, autophagy, where the body cleans itself out and makes new cells, and we mentioned that IF triggers autophagy. Someone who hasn't read the literature will not know this, but the truth is, there is no point where your body is not working even in the middle of the night. When we fast, we help the body divert its attention from continually digesting food to working on other essential processes, and this is one of the great things about practicing IF.

The Brain Needs a Constant Supply of Glucose

This comes from those who think that your brain can only use glucose for fuel, but now that we are almost at the end of this book, you know this is not true. We introduced the term *ketosis* earlier in this book, where we described this process as the point where your body switches from burning glycogen to burning fat as it goes into ketosis due to the liver producing ketones. Ketones provide fuel for your brain during fasting periods, so no, your body does not need a constant supply of glucose to function.

Breakfast Is the Most Important Meal of the Day

Proponents of this myth believe in the old mindset that you cannot skip breakfast as it is the *most important meal of the day*. These are people who believe that breakfast must be scheduled within the first couple of hours of starting your day. These people also believe that skipping breakfast slows down your metabolism, something that research has proven is not true (Moro et al., 2016). Other people believe that skipping breakfast will trigger a binge later since you will be starving then. This is also not supported by research (Horne et al., 2015), and as I have mentioned in earlier chapters, one of the goals of IF is to help you build good habits around food. Scheduling breakfast a little bit later in the day is not going to rob you of the important nutrition that comes from eating eggs and other *breakfast* foods; however, it may allow you the added advantage of participating in family dinners during your evenings.

IF Puts You in Starvation Mode

IF does not put you in starvation mode, but rather, it allows the body to take a break from digesting food, to work on other processes, such as cell regeneration. If you remember, during the hunter-gatherer times, people went for long periods of not eating, and the human body was and is still adapted to this.

IF Will Cause a Dangerous Drop in Blood Levels

One of the main benefits of IF is how it helps in the regulation of insulin levels. Many studies, some of which we discussed in the early chapters, demonstrated the significant role that IF plays in improving insulin resistance and reversing the symptoms of type 2 diabetes. When IF was tested among patients with type 2 diabetes, some of them ended up terminating their insulin therapy because they regained control of their insulin levels (Furmli, et al., 2018).

IF Will Cause You to Lose Muscle

We discussed in the chapter on combining IF with exercise that even though some studies showed that those who combined IF with strength training did not gain muscle compared to those who were not on IF, research shows that they did not lose it either (Moro et al., 2016). IF has another positive *side effect* for those who are into bodybuilding, and that is the fact that it boosts the production of HGH, which has great benefits for building bones and tissue in our bodies. It also helps them maintain a low body fat percentage.

IF Is Not Good for Your Health

This could not be further from the truth. In the first chapter of this book, we discussed the many health benefits that IF presents, such as improved insulin sensitivity, antiaging, increased longevity, prevention of certain cancers, lowering your risk of degenerative diseases such as Alzheimer's, and boosting the production of BDNF which protects you against depression and other mental health conditions. These are over and above the fat-burning effects of IF.

IF Is the Magic Bullet

I would like to end this chapter by discussing this popular myth. This is certainly not true. IF is not the magic bullet that fixes everything overnight. When combined with exercise and healthy eating habits, IF will deliver great health benefits for you, but it is not the magic bullet; it works when you do your part. You will also have to maintain healthy eating habits throughout your life. By the way, no diet out there is the magic bullet, and to believe that will be to set yourself up for failure.

I hope I have addressed most of the myths you have heard about IF in this chapter. Now, it's up to you to do your part and educate others next time you hear someone saying something that is not true about IF.

Conclusion

You'll never change your life until you change something you do daily. The secret of your success is found in your daily routine.

— John C. Maxwell

Now that we've come to the end of this book, I wanted to share this quote with you. In your hands, you have a powerful tool that will guide you every step of the way on your IF journey. By purchasing a copy of this book, you already took the first step toward changing what you do daily. The next step is obviously using the book. That is not to say that this book is all you will ever need. By all means, do consult other resources to supplement the information given here. But in this book, we have attempted to answer almost any question that someone who is starting IF may have.

Here is a summary of what you would have learned from this book:

In Chapter 1, we introduced you to the different IF plans and described each one, how it works and what its health benefits are to give you a general sense of how the individual plans differ. This was to present you with as much information as possible to help you get a sense of which plan you may want to try based on your specific needs and your lifestyle.

In Chapter 2, we discussed IF in relation to women, specifically, the advantages and disadvantages that this diet may present for women. With that in mind, Chapter 3 drilled down to what plan(s) may be more suitable for you based on the information given in the first two chapters.

In Chapter 4, we discussed the sensitive issue of age, specifically what unique health problems people who are 50 and above face, and what IF can or cannot do for you at this age. Up to this point, we were really helping you decide if IF is for you or not, with emphasis on seeking medical counsel if you are not sure.

After Chapter 5, we got into the practical stuff, what to eat and what to look out for in selecting your food. We also helped you with the tools to get you started in Chapter 6, whether to incorporate exercise or not (Chapter 7), and we presented examples of meal plans and recipes in Chapters 8 and 9. In the last chapter (Chapter 10), we addressed and hopefully dispelled some of the myths around IF.

So What Are the Key *Take-Home* Lessons?

- IF is not just about skipping meals; it's about how you structure your meals and schedule your meals to reap the maximum benefits from *what* and *when* you eat.
- IF has many plans, and you should choose a plan that addresses your health concerns and one that is easy to incorporate into your lifestyle.
- IF delivers many health benefits: It increases fat burning due to ketosis which results in weight loss, improves your heart health and brain health, and prevents or reduces the risk of certain degenerative diseases like Parkinson's and Alzheimer's, certain cancers, and type 2 diabetes.

- Even though most people think you can eat whatever you like on IF, this does not mean eating junk food. In this book, we strongly encouraged healthy choices and keeping an eye on your calorie intake. IF should not be about eating boring food. You can create interesting meals, as shown in Chapters 8 and 9, and yes, you can still have a slice of cake or a slice of pizza.
- Combining IF with a training schedule has the potential to double your weight loss efforts. Exercising on an empty stomach increases fat burning because it takes advantage of the already low glycogen stores in your body.
- Starting slowly, with a healthy and positive mindset, will set you up for success. Choosing a plan like the Crescendo method will ease you into a fasting routine, and as you develop your *fasting muscle*, you can increase your fasting hours and move on to other plans.
- Not sure if you are the best candidate for IF? Consult your healthcare provider. IF is not for everyone, so please make sure that you don't fall under the groups that IF is not recommended for. Those groups are listed in various sections throughout this book.

Leave a Review

As an independent author with a small marketing budget, reviews are my livelihood on this platform. If you enjoyed this book, I'd really appreciate it if you left your honest feedback. You can do this by clicking the link below. I love hearing from my readers and I personally read every single review.

https://www.amazon.com/review/create-review/?
asin=B0BSTL5G7R

References

Abdellatif, M., & Sedej, S. (2020). Cardiovascular benefits of intermittent fasting. *Cardiovascular Research, 116*(3), e36–e38. https://doi.org/10.1093/cvr/cvaa022

Aghayev, R. (n.d.). *Eating junk while intermittent fasting: Can you eat whatever you want?* IFIT Zone. https://ifitzone.ca/eating-junk-while-intermittent-fasting/

Alirezaei, M., Kemball, C. C., Flynn, C. T., Wood, M. R., Whitton, J. L., & Kiosses, W. B. (2010). Short-term fasting induces profound neuronal autophagy. *Autophagy, 6*(6), 702–710. https://doi.org/10.4161/auto.6.6.12376

Allrecipes | Food, friends, and recipe inspiration. (2019). Allrecipes. https://www.allrecipes.com/

American Cancer Society. (n.d.). *Global cancer facts & figures.* https://www.cancer.org/research/cancer-facts-statistics/global.html

Anson, R. M., Guo, Z., de Cabo, R., Iyun, T., Rios, M., Hagepanos, A., Ingram, D. K., Lane, M. A., & Mattson, M. P. (2003). Intermittent fasting dissociates beneficial effects of dietary restriction on glucose metabolism and neuronal resistance to injury from calorie intake. *Proceedings of the National Academy of Sciences, 100*(10), 6216–6220. https://doi.org/10.1073/pnas.1035720100

Anton, S. D., Moehl, K., Donahoo, W. T., Marosi, K., Lee, S. A., Mainous, A. G., Leeuwenburgh, C., & Mattson, M. P. (2018). Flipping the Metabolic Switch: Understanding and Applying the Health Benefits of Fasting. *Obesity (Silver Spring, Md.), 26*(2), 254–268. https://doi.org/10.1002/oby.22065

Antoni, R., Johnston, K., Collins, A., & Robertson, M. D. (2014). The Effects of Intermittent Energy Restriction on Indices of Cardiometabolic Health. *Research in Endocrinology*, 1–24. https://doi.org/10.5171/2014.459119

Arnason, T. G., Bowen, M. W., & Mansell, K. D. (2017). Effects of intermittent fasting on health markers in those with type 2 diabetes: A pilot study. *World Journal of Diabetes, 8*(4), 154. https://doi.org/10.4239/wjd.v8.i4.154

Asgary, S., Rastqar, A., & Keshvari, M. (2018). Functional Food and Cardiovascular Disease Prevention and Treatment: A Review. *Journal of the American College of Nutrition, 37*(5), 429–455. https://doi.org/10.1080/07315724.2017.1410867

Baik, S. H., Rajeev, V., Fann, D. Y.-W., Jo, D.-G., & Arumugam, T. V. (2020). Intermittent fasting increases adult hippocampal neurogenesis. *Brain and Behavior, 10*(1), e01444. https://doi.org/10.1002/brb3.1444

Barnosky, A. R., Hoddy, K. K., Unterman, T. G., & Varady, K. A. (2014a). Intermittent fasting vs daily calorie restriction for type 2 diabetes prevention: a review of human findings. *Translational Research, 164*(4), 302–311. https://doi.org/10.1016/j.trsl.2014.05.013

Barnosky, A. R., Hoddy, K. K., Unterman, T. G., & Varady, K. A. (2014b). Intermittent fasting vs daily calorie restriction for type 2 diabetes prevention: a review of human findings. *Translational Research, 164*(4), 302–311. https://doi.org/10.1016/j.trsl.2014.05.013

Bartholomew, C. L., Muhlestein, J. B., May, H. T., Le, V. T., Galenko, O., Garrett, K. D., Brunker, C., Hopkins, R. O., Carlquist, J. F., Knowlton, K. U., Anderson, J. L., Bailey, B. W., & Horne, B. D. (2021). Randomized controlled trial of once-per-week intermittent fasting for health improvement: the WONDERFUL trial. *European Heart Journal Open, 1*(2). https://doi.org/10.1093/ehjopen/oeab026

Benefits of intermittent fasting for women over 50. (2022, March 12). Primewomen. https://primewomen.com/health/nutrition/benefits-of-intermittent-fasting-for-women-over-50/#:~:text=Most%20older%20women%20find%20a

Bhutani, S., Klempel, M. C., Kroeger, C. M., Trepanowski, J. F., & Varady, K. A. (2013). Alternate day fasting and endurance exercise combine to reduce body weight and favorably alter plasma lipids in obese humans. *Obesity, 21*(7), 1370–1379. https://doi.org/10.1002/oby.20353

Bjarnadottir, A. (2018, May 31). *The beginner's guide to the 5:2 diet.* Healthline. https://www.healthline.com/nutrition/the-5-2-diet-guide#TOC_TITLE_HDR_3

Bjarnadottir, A., & Kubala, J. (2020, August 4). *Alternate-day fasting: A comprehensive beginner's guide.* Healthline. https://www.healthline.com/nutrition/alternate-day-fasting-guide#weight-loss

Björkholm, C., & Monteggia, L. M. (2016). BDNF – a key transducer of antidepressant effects. *Neuropharmacology, 102*, 72–79. https://doi.org/10.1016/j.neuropharm.2015.10.034

Blanchet, C., Lucas, M., Julien, P., Morin, R., Gingras, S., & Dewailly, É. (2005). Fatty acid composition of wild and farmed Atlantic salmon (Salmo salar) and rainbow trout (Oncorhynchus mykiss). *Lipids, 40*(5), 529–531. https://doi.org/10.1007/s11745-005-1414-0

Blekkenhorst, L., Sim, M., Bondonno, C., Bondonno, N., Ward, N., Prince, R., Devine, A., Lewis, J., & Hodgson, J. (2018). Cardiovascular Health Benefits of Specific Vegetable Types: A Narrative Review. *Nutrients, 10*(5), 595. https://doi.org/10.3390/nu10050595

Blesso, C., N., & Luz Fernandez, M. (2018). Dietary Cholesterol, Serum Lipids, and Heart Disease: Are Eggs Working for or Against You? *Nutrients, 10*(4), 426. https://doi.org/10.3390/nu10040426

Bolling, B. W., Chen, C.-Y. O., McKay, D. L., & Blumberg, J. B. (2011). Tree nut phytochemicals: composition, antioxidant capacity, bioactivity, impact factors. A systematic review of almonds, Brazils, cashews, hazelnuts, macadamias, pecans, pine nuts, pistachios and walnuts. *Nutrition Research Reviews, 24*(2), 244–275. https://doi.org/10.1017/s095442241100014x

Brennan, D. (2021, September 27). *What to know about intermittent fasting for women after 50.* WebMD. https://www.webmd.com/healthy-aging/what-to-know-about-intermittent-fasting-for-women-after-50#091e9c5e821476b0-2-6

Brill, J. B. (2021, March 24). *10 myths about intermittent fasting debunked.* Dummies. https://www.dummies.com/article/body-mind-spirit/physical-health-well-being/diet-nutrition/intermittent-fasting/10-myths-about-intermittent-fasting-debunked-275829/

Brooks, A. (2020, May 13). *15 superfoods and the scientific reasons to eat them.* Everyday Health. https://www.everydayhealth.com/photogallery/superfoods.aspx

Buijsse, B., Feskens, E. J. M., Kok, F. J., & Kromhout, D. (2006). Cocoa Intake, Blood Pressure, and Cardiovascular Mortality.

Archives of Internal Medicine, *166*(4), 411. https://doi.org/10.1001/archinte.166.4.411

Byrne, N. M., Sainsbury, A., King, N. A., Hills, A. P., & Wood, R. E. (2017). Intermittent energy restriction improves weight loss efficiency in obese men: the MATADOR study. *International Journal of Obesity*, *42*(2), 129–138. https://doi.org/10.1038/ijo.2017.206

Calorie calculator. (n.d.). Calculator.net. https://www.calculator.net/calorie-calculator.html

Caporuscio, J. (2019, September 6). *Keto flu: What it is, symptoms, and home remedies*. Medical News Today. https://www.medicalnewstoday.com/articles/326276

Carter, S., Clifton, P. M., & Keogh, J. B. (2018). Effect of Intermittent Compared With Continuous Energy Restricted Diet on Glycemic Control in Patients With Type 2 Diabetes. *JAMA Network Open*, *1*(3), e180756. https://doi.org/10.1001/jamanetworkopen.2018.0756

Catenacci, V. A., Pan, Z., Ostendorf, D., Brannon, S., Gozansky, W. S., Mattson, M. P., Martin, B., MacLean, P. S., Melanson, E. L., & Troy Donahoo, W. (2016). A randomized pilot study comparing zero-calorie alternate-day fasting to daily caloric restriction in adults with obesity. *Obesity*, *24*(9), 1874–1883. https://doi.org/10.1002/oby.21581

Catterson, J. H., Khericha, M., Dyson, M. C., Vincent, A. J., Callard, R., Haveron, S. M., Rajasingam, A., Ahmad, M., & Partridge, L. (2018). Short-Term, Intermittent Fasting Induces Long-Lasting Gut Health and TOR-Independent Lifespan Extension. *Current Biology*, *28*(11), 1714-1724.e4. https://doi.org/10.1016/j.cub.2018.04.015

CDC. (2020a, January 31). *LDL and HDL cholesterol: "Bad" and "good" cholesterol.* https://www.cdc.gov/cholesterol/ldl_hdl.htm#:~:text=LDL%20(low%2Ddensity%20lipoprotein)

CDC. (2020b, February 25). *Facts about hypertension.* https://www.cdc.gov/bloodpressure/facts.htm#:~:text=Nearly%20half%20of%20adults%20in

CDC. (2021, February 11). *Adult obesity facts.* https://www.cdc.gov/obesity/data/adult.html

CDC. (2022a, June 3). *Planning meals.* https://www.cdc.gov/healthyweight/healthy_eating/meals.html

CDC. (2022b, September 6). *FastStats - Overweight prevalence.* https://www.cdc.gov/nchs/fastats/obesity-overweight.htm

Christiansen, S. (2022, May 27). *Diabetes and intermittent fasting.* Verywell Health. https://www.verywellhealth.com/diabetes-and-intermittent-fasting-4844452#toc-types-of-if-diets-for-diabetes

Cienfuegos, S., Corapi, S., Gabel, K., Ezpeleta, M., Kalam, F., Lin, S., Pavlou, V., & Varady, K. A. (2022). Effect of Intermittent Fasting on Reproductive Hormone Levels in Females and Males: A Review of Human Trials. *Nutrients, 14*(11), 2343. https://doi.org/10.3390/nu14112343

Cienfuegos, S., Gabel, K., Kalam, F., Ezpeleta, M., Lin, S., & Varady, K. A. (2021). Changes in body weight and metabolic risk during time restricted feeding in premenopausal versus postmenopausal women. *Experimental Gerontology, 154,* 111545. https://doi.org/10.1016/j.exger.2021.111545

Cleveland HeartLab. (2021, July 21). *Intermittent fasting: A new way to help your heart and your health.* https://www.clevelandheartlab.com/blog/intermittent-fasting-a-new-way-to-help-your-heart-and-your-health/#:~:text=Intermittent%20fasting%20has%20a%20lot

Cole, W. (2021, December 30). *Intermittent fasting meal plan: Here's exactly when & what to eat.* MindBodyGreen. https://www.mindbodygreen.com/articles/intermittent-fasting-diet-plan-how-to-schedule-meals

Coyle, D. (2018, July 22). *Intermittent fasting for women: A beginner's guide.* Healthline. https://www.healthline.com/nutrition/intermittent-fasting-for-women#safety-and-side-effects

Crescendo fasting for women. (2019, February 4). Konscious Keto. https://konsciousketo.com/blogs/keto/crescendo-fasting

Crescendo fasting: The best fasting method for women to get quick results. (2022, July 14). Fit Girls for Life. https://www.fitgirls4life.com/crescendo-fasting/#tve-jump-173db410ee7

Crozier, S. J., Preston, A. G., Hurst, J. W., Payne, M. J., Mann, J., Hainly, L., & Miller, D. L. (2011). Cacao seeds are a "Super Fruit": A comparative analysis of various fruit powders and products. *Chemistry Central Journal, 5*(1), 5. https://doi.org/10.1186/1752-153x-5-5

Dady, J. (2021, March 22). *5:2 diet meal plans: What to eat for 500 calorie fast days.* GoodtoKnow. https://www.goodto.com/food/5-2-diet-meal-plans-what-to-eat-for-500-calorie-fast-days-108045

Davis, L. M., Pauly, J. R., Readnower, R. D., Rho, J. M., & Sullivan, P. G. (2008). Fasting is neuroprotective following traumatic brain injury. *Journal of Neuroscience Research, 86*(8), 1812–1822. https://doi.org/10.1002/jnr.21628

de Cabo, R., & Mattson, M. P. (2019). Effects of Intermittent Fasting on Health, Aging, and Disease. *New England Journal of Medicine, 381*(26), 2541–2551. https://doi.org/10.1056/nejmra1905136

de la Fuente-Arrillaga, C., Martinez-Gonzalez, M. A., Zazpe, I., Vazquez-Ruiz, Z., Benito-Corchon, S., & Bes-Rastrollo, M. (2014). Glycemic load, glycemic index, bread and incidence of overweight/obesity in a Mediterranean cohort: the SUN project. *BMC Public Health, 14*(1). https://doi.org/10.1186/1471-2458-14-1091

Devore, E. E., Kang, J. H., Breteler, M. M. B., & Grodstein, F. (2012). Dietary intakes of berries and flavonoids in relation to cognitive decline. *Annals of Neurology, 72*(1), 135–143. https://doi.org/10.1002/ana.23594

Dhaka, V., Gulia, N., Ahlawat, K. S., & Khatkar, B. S. (2011). Trans fats—sources, health risks and alternative approach - A review. *Journal of Food Science and Technology, 48*(5), 534–541. https://doi.org/10.1007/s13197-010-0225-8

Dhillon, K. K., & Gupta, S. (2022, February 10). *Biochemistry, ketogenesis*. National Library of Medicine. https://www.ncbi.nlm.nih.gov/books/NBK493179/

Domaszewski, P., Konieczny, M., Pakosz, P., Bączkowicz, D., & Sadowska-Krępa, E. (2020). Effect of a Six-Week Intermittent Fasting Intervention Program on the Composition of the Human Body in Women over 60 Years of Age. *International Journal of Environmental Research and Public Health, 17*(11), 4138. https://doi.org/10.3390/ijerph17114138

Dong, T. A., Sandesara, P. B., Dhindsa, D. S., Mehta, A., Arneson, L. C., Dollar, A. L., Taub, P. R., & Sperling, L. S. (2020). Intermittent Fasting: A Heart Healthy Dietary Pattern? *The American Journal of Medicine, 133*(8). https://doi.org/10.1016/j.amjmed.2020.03.030

Dornbush, S., & Aeddula, N. R. (2022, April 14). *Physiology, leptin*. National Library of Medicine. https://www.ncbi.nlm.nih.gov/books/NBK537038/

Du, H., Li, L., Bennett, D., Guo, Y., Turnbull, I., Yang, L., Bragg, F., Bian, Z., Chen, Y., Chen, J., Millwood, I. Y., Sansome, S., Ma, L., Huang, Y., Zhang, N., Zheng, X., Sun, Q., Key, T. J., Collins, R., &

Peto, R. (2017). Fresh fruit consumption in relation to incident diabetes and diabetic vascular complications: A 7-y prospective study of 0.5 million Chinese adults. *PLoS Medicine, 14*(4). https://doi.org/10.1371/journal.pmed.1002279

Du, L., Hickey, R. W., Bayir, H., Watkins, S. C., Tyurin, V. A., Guo, F., Kochanek, P. M., Jenkins, L. W., Ren, J., Gibson, G., Chu, C. T., Kagan, V. E., & Clark, R. S. B. (2009). Starving Neurons Show Sex Difference in Autophagy*. *Journal of Biological Chemistry, 284*(4), 2383–2396. https://doi.org/10.1074/jbc.M804396200

Eat stop eat reviews: Does it work for actual customer results? (2022, February 11). Vashon-Maury Island Beachcomber. https://www.vashonbeachcomber.com/national-marketplace/eat-stop-eat-reviews-does-it-work-for-actual-customer-results/

Elavsky, S., & McAuley, E. (2007). Physical activity and mental health outcomes during menopause: A randomized controlled trial. *Annals of Behavioral Medicine, 33*(2), 132–142. https://doi.org/10.1007/bf02879894

English, N. (2019, June 7). *Does intermittent fasting affect women differently than men?* BarBend. https://barbend.com/intermittent-fasting-women/

Eshghinia, S., & Mohammadzadeh, F. (2013). The effects of modified alternate-day fasting diet on weight loss and CAD risk factors in overweight and obese women. *Journal of Diabetes & Metabolic Disorders, 12*(1), 4. https://doi.org/10.1186/2251-6581-12-4

Faris, M. A.-I. E., Kacimi, S., Al-Kurd, R. A., Fararjeh, M. A., Bustanji, Y. K., Mohammad, M. K., & Salem, M. L. (2012). Intermittent fasting during Ramadan attenuates proinflammatory cytokines and immune cells in healthy subjects. *Nutrition Research, 32*(12), 947–955. https://doi.org/10.1016/j.nutres.2012.06.021

Fissler, P., Küster, O. C., Laptinskaya, D., Loy, L. S., von Arnim, C. A. F., & Kolassa, I.-T. (2018). Jigsaw Puzzling Taps Multiple Cognitive Abilities and Is a Potential Protective Factor for Cognitive Aging. *Frontiers in Aging Neuroscience, 10.* https://doi.org/10.3389/fnagi.2018.00299

Fitzgerald, K. C., Vizthum, D., Henry-Barron, B., Schweitzer, A., Cassard, S. D., Kossoff, E., Hartman, A. L., Kapogiannis, D., Sullivan, P., Baer, D. J., Mattson, M. P., Appel, L. J., & Mowry, E. M. (2018). Effect of intermittent vs. daily calorie restriction on changes in weight and patient-reported outcomes in people with multiple sclerosis. *Multiple Sclerosis and Related Disorders, 23,* 33–39. https://doi.org/10.1016/j.msard.2018.05.002

5:2 diet recipes. (n.d.). BBC Good Food. https://www.bbcgoodfood.com/recipes/collection/5-2-recipes

Fletcher, J. (2019, April 5). *Intermittent fasting for weight loss: 5 tips to start.* Medical News Today. https://www.medicalnewstoday.com/articles/324882

Fluid and electrolyte balance. (2021, November 19). MedlinePlus. https://medlineplus.gov/fluidandelectrolytebalance.html#:~:text=Electrolytes%20are%20minerals%20in%20your

Foster, D. W., & McGarry, J. D. (2008). The Regulation of Ketogenesis. *Ciba Foundation Symposium 87 - Metabolic Acidosis,* 120–144. https://doi.org/10.1002/9780470720691.ch7

Frey, M. (2020, September 30). *Pros and cons of intermittent fasting.* Verywell Fit. https://www.verywellfit.com/intermittent-fasting-pros-and-cons-4688805

Fulgoni, V. L., Dreher, M., & Davenport, A. J. (2013). Avocado consumption is associated with better diet quality and nutrient intake, and lower metabolic syndrome risk in US adults: results from the National Health and Nutrition Examination Survey (NHANES)

160   *References*

2001–2008. *Nutrition Journal, 12*(1). https://doi.org/10.1186/1475-2891-12-1

Furmli, S., Elmasry, R., Ramos, M., & Fung, J. (2018). Therapeutic use of intermittent fasting for people with type 2 diabetes as an alternative to insulin. *BMJ Case Reports*, bcr-2017-221854. https://doi.org/10.1136/bcr-2017-221854

Glick, D., Barth, S., & Macleod, K. F. (2010). Autophagy: cellular and molecular mechanisms. *The Journal of Pathology, 221*(1), 3–12. https://doi.org/10.1002/path.2697

Goodrick, C. L., Ingram, D. K., Reynolds, M. A., Freeman, J. R., & Cider, N. L. (1982). Effects of intermittent feeding upon growth and life span in rats. *Gerontology, 28*(4), 233–241. https://doi.org/10.1159/000212538

Gotthardt, J. D., Verpeut, J. L., Yeomans, B. L., Yang, J. A., Yasrebi, A., Roepke, T. A., & Bello, N. T. (2016). Intermittent Fasting Promotes Fat Loss With Lean Mass Retention, Increased Hypothalamic Norepinephrine Content, and Increased Neuropeptide Y Gene Expression in Diet-Induced Obese Male Mice. *Endocrinology, 157*(2), 679–691. https://doi.org/10.1210/en.2015-1622

Govers, C., Berkel Kasikci, M., van der Sluis, A. A., & Mes, J. J. (2017). Review of the health effects of berries and their phytochemicals on the digestive and immune systems. *Nutrition Reviews, 76*(1), 29–46. https://doi.org/10.1093/nutrit/nux039

Grajower, M. M., & Horne, B. D. (2019). Clinical Management of Intermittent Fasting in Patients with Diabetes Mellitus. *Nutrients, 11*(4), 873. https://doi.org/10.3390/nu11040873

Gunnars, K. (2021, May 13). *10 evidence-based health benefits of intermittent fasting*. Healthline. https://www.healthline.-

com/nutrition/10-health-benefits-of-intermittent-fasting#TOC_TITLE_HDR_3

Halagappa, V. K. M., Guo, Z., Pearson, M., Matsuoka, Y., Cutler, R. G., Laferla, F. M., & Mattson, M. P. (2007). Intermittent fasting and caloric restriction ameliorate age-related behavioral deficits in the triple-transgenic mouse model of Alzheimer's disease. *Neurobiology of Disease, 26*(1), 212–220. https://doi.org/10.1016/j.nbd.2006.12.019

Hanka, S. (2021, July 2). *10 intermittent fasting benefits and potential risks*. Trifecta. https://www.trifectanutrition.-com/blog/intermittent-fasting-benefits-and-potential-risks

Hardick, B. J. (2019, May 1). *7 intermittent fasting mistakes that could make you gain weight*. MindBodyGreen. https://www.mind-bodygreen.com/articles/intermittent-fasting-mistakes-that-could-make-you-gain-weight/

Hartman, M. L., Veldhuis, J. D., Johnson, M. L., Lee, M. M., Alberti, K. G., Samojlik, E., & Thorner, M. O. (1992). Augmented growth hormone (GH) secretory burst frequency and amplitude mediate enhanced GH secretion during a two-day fast in normal men. *The Journal of Clinical Endocrinology and Metabolism, 74*(4), 757–765. https://doi.org/10.1210/jcem.74.4.1548337

Harvard Health Publishing. (2021a, February 15). *Belly fat may pose more danger for women than for men*. https://www.health.har-vard.edu/womens-health/belly-fat-may-pose-more-danger-for-women-than-for-men

Harvard Health Publishing. (2021b, February 28). *Intermittent fasting: The positive news continues*. https://www.health.harvard.e-du/blog/intermittent-fasting-surprising-update-2018062914156

Harvard T.H. Chan School of Public Health. (2012, September 18). *Nuts for the heart.* https://www.hsph.harvard.edu/nutrition-source/nuts-for-the-heart/

Harvard T.H. Chan School of Public Health. (2018, September 25). *Whole grains.* https://www.hsph.harvard.edu/nutritionsource/what-should-you-eat/whole-grains/

Harvie, M. N., Pegington, M., Mattson, M. P., Frystyk, J., Dillon, B., Evans, G., Cuzick, J., Jebb, S. A., Martin, B., Cutler, R. G., Son, T. G., Maudsley, S., Carlson, O. D., Egan, J. M., Flyvbjerg, A., & Howell, A. (2010). The effects of intermittent or continuous energy restriction on weight loss and metabolic disease risk markers: a randomized trial in young overweight women. *International Journal of Obesity*, *35*(5), 714–727. https://doi.org/10.1038/ijo.2010.171

Harvie, M., & Howell, A. (2017). Potential Benefits and Harms of Intermittent Energy Restriction and Intermittent Fasting Amongst Obese, Overweight and Normal Weight Subjects—A Narrative Review of Human and Animal Evidence. *Behavioral Sciences*, *7*(4), 4. https://doi.org/10.3390/bs7010004

Healthy eating archives. (2020, November 30). Zulusingleandfab. https://zulusingleandfab.com/category/healthy-eating/

Heilbronn, L. K., Civitarese, A. E., Bogacka, I., Smith, S. R., Hulver, M., & Ravussin, E. (2005). Glucose Tolerance and Skeletal Muscle Gene Expression in Response to Alternate Day Fasting. *Obesity Research*, *13*(3), 574–581. https://doi.org/10.1038/oby.2005.61

Heilbronn, L. K., Smith, S. R., Martin, C. K., Anton, S. D., & Ravussin, E. (2005). Alternate-day fasting in nonobese subjects: effects on body weight, body composition, and energy metabolism. *The American Journal of Clinical Nutrition*, *81*(1), 69–73. https://doi.org/10.1093/ajcn/81.1.69

Hill, A. (2022, June 14). *Eat stop eat review: Does it work for weight loss?* Healthline. https://www.healthline.com/nutrition/eat-stop-eat-review#basics

Hisatomi, Y., & Kugino, K. (2019). Changes in bone density and bone quality caused by single fasting for 96 hours in rats. *PeerJ, 6,* e6161. https://doi.org/10.7717/peerj.6161

Ho, K. Y., Veldhuis, J. D., Johnson, M. L., Furlanetto, R., Evans, W. S., Alberti, K. G., & Thorner, M. O. (1988). Fasting enhances growth hormone secretion and amplifies the complex rhythms of growth hormone secretion in man. *Journal of Clinical Investigation, 81*(4), 968–975. https://www.ncbi.nlm.nih.gov/pmc/articles/PMC329619/

Hoddy, K. K., Gibbons, C., Kroeger, C. M., Trepanowski, J. F., Barnosky, A., Bhutani, S., Gabel, K., Finlayson, G., & Varady, K. A. (2016). Changes in hunger and fullness in relation to gut peptides before and after 8 weeks of alternate day fasting. *Clinical Nutrition, 35*(6), 1380–1385. https://doi.org/10.1016/j.clnu.2016.03.011

Hoddy, K. K., Kroeger, C. M., Trepanowski, J. F., Barnosky, A., Bhutani, S., & Varady, K. A. (2014). Meal timing during alternate day fasting: Impact on body weight and cardiovascular disease risk in obese adults. *Obesity,* n/a-n/a. https://doi.org/10.1002/oby.20909

Horne, B. D., Muhlestein, J. B., & Anderson, J. L. (2015). Health effects of intermittent fasting: hormesis or harm? A systematic review. *The American Journal of Clinical Nutrition, 102*(2), 464–470. https://doi.org/10.3945/ajcn.115.109553

Hussin, N. M., Shahar, S., Teng, N. I. M. F., Ngah, W. Z. W., & Das, S. K. (2013). Efficacy of Fasting and Calorie Restriction (FCR) on mood and depression among ageing men. *The Journal of Nutrition, Health & Aging, 17*(8), 674–680. https://doi.org/10.1007/s12603-013-0344-9

Ibrahim Abdalla, M. M. (2015). Ghrelin – Physiological Functions and Regulation. *European Endocrinology, 11*(2), 90–95. https://doi.org/10.17925/EE.2015.11.02.90

ISSA. (2022, April 1). *Intermittent fasting: Women vs. men.* https://www.issaonline.com/blog/post/this-hot-diet-trend-is-not-recommended-for-women

Iturria-Medina, Y., Sotero, R. C., Toussaint, P. J., Mateos-Pérez, J. M., & Evans, A. C. (2016). Early role of vascular dysregulation on late-onset Alzheimer's disease based on multifactorial data-driven analysis. *Nature Communications, 7*(1). https://doi.org/10.1038/ncomms11934

Jamshed, H., Beyl, R. A., Della Manna, D. L., Yang, E. S., Ravussin, E., & Peterson, C. M. (2019). Early Time-Restricted Feeding Improves 24-Hour Glucose Levels and Affects Markers of the Circadian Clock, Aging, and Autophagy in Humans. *Nutrients, 11*(6), 1234. https://doi.org/10.3390/nu11061234

Jarreau, P. (2020, October 6). *Your menstrual cycle on intermittent fasting.* LIFE Apps. https://lifeapps.io/fasting/your-menstrual-cycle-on-intermittent-fasting/

Jaspers, R. T., Zillikens, M. C., Friesema, E. C. H., Paoli, G., Bloch, W., Uitterlinden, A. G., Goglia, F., Lanni, A., & Lange, P. (2016). Exercise, fasting, and mimetics: toward beneficial combinations? *The FASEB Journal, 31*(1), 14–28. https://doi.org/10.1096/fj.201600652r

Jockers. (2019, March 22). *Crescendo fasting: The best fasting strategy for women?* DrJockers.com. https://drjockers.com/crescendo-fasting/

John C. Maxwell quote. (n.d.). Quotefancy. https://quotefancy.com/quote/840994/John-C-Maxwell-You-will-never-change-your-life-until-you-change-something-you-do-daily

Johnson, J. B., Laub, D. R., & John, S. (2006). The effect on health of alternate day calorie restriction: Eating less and more than needed on alternate days prolongs life. *Medical Hypotheses, 67*(2), 209–211. https://doi.org/10.1016/j.mehy.2006.01.030

Kale: Rich in antioxidants. (2021, April 6). American Institute for Cancer Research. https://www.aicr.org/cancer-prevention/food-facts/dark-green-leafy-vegetables/

Kerksick, C. M., Arent, S., Schoenfeld, B. J., Stout, J. R., Campbell, B., Wilborn, C. D., Taylor, L., Kalman, D., Smith-Ryan, A. E., Kreider, R. B., Willoughby, D., Arciero, P. J., VanDusseldorp, T. A., Ormsbee, M. J., Wildman, R., Greenwood, M., Ziegenfuss, T. N., Aragon, A. A., & Antonio, J. (2017). International society of sports nutrition position stand: nutrient timing. *Journal of the International Society of Sports Nutrition, 14*(1). https://doi.org/10.1186/s12970-017-0189-4

Kerndt, P. R., Naughton, J. L., Driscoll, C. E., & Loxterkamp, D. A. (1982). Fasting: The History, Pathophysiology and Complications. *Western Journal of Medicine, 137*(5), 379–399. https://www.ncbi.nlm.nih.gov/pmc/articles/PMC1274154/?page=2

Kerti, L., Witte, A. V., Winkler, A., Grittner, U., Rujescu, D., & Floel, A. (2013). Higher glucose levels associated with lower memory and reduced hippocampal microstructure. *Neurology, 81*(20), 1746–1752. https://doi.org/10.1212/01.wnl.0000435561.00234.ee

Kim, Y., Kim, S., Kim, C., Sato, T., Kojima, M., & Park, S. (2015). Ghrelin is required for dietary restriction-induced enhancement of hippocampal neurogenesis: lessons from ghrelin knockout mice. *Endocrine Journal, 62*(3), 269–275. https://doi.org/10.1507/endocrj.ej14-0436

Koushali, A. N., Hajiamini, Z., Ebadi, A., Bayat, N., & Khamseh, F. (2013). Effect of Ramadan fasting on emotional reactions in nurses.

Iranian Journal of Nursing and Midwifery Research, 18(3), 232–236. https://www.ncbi.nlm.nih.gov/pmc/articles/PMC3748544/

Kubala, J. (2018, July 3). *The warrior diet: Review and beginner's guide.* Healthline. https://www.healthline.com/nutrition/warrior-diet-guide#benefits

Kumar, S., & Kaur, G. (2013). Intermittent Fasting Dietary Restriction Regimen Negatively Influences Reproduction in Young Rats: A Study of Hypothalamo-Hypophysial-Gonadal Axis. *PLoS ONE, 8*(1), e52416. https://doi.org/10.1371/journal.pone.0052416

Lederer, S. (2022, August 2). *Crescendo fasting method: Is it the best plan for women?* Mental Food Chain. https://www.mentalfoodchain.com/crescendo-fasting-method/

Lee, C., Raffaghello, L., Brandhorst, S., Safdie, F. M., Bianchi, G., Martin-Montalvo, A., Pistoia, V., Wei, M., Hwang, S., Merlino, A., Emionite, L., de Cabo, R., & Longo, V. D. (2012). Fasting cycles retard growth of tumors and sensitize a range of cancer cell types to chemotherapy. *Science Translational Medicine, 4*(124), 124ra27. https://doi.org/10.1126/scitranslmed.3003293

Leech, J. (2017, June 3). *10 delicious herbs and spices with powerful health benefits.* Healthline. https://www.healthline.com/nutrition/10-healthy-herbs-and-spices#TOC_TITLE_HDR_3

Leonard, J. (2020, January 17). *A guide to 16:8 intermittent fasting.* Medical News Today. https://www.medicalnewstoday.com/articles/327398#side-effects-and-risks

Li, L., Wang, Z., & Zuo, Z. (2013). Chronic intermittent fasting improves cognitive functions and brain structures in mice. *PloS One, 8*(6), e66069. https://doi.org/10.1371/journal.pone.0066069

Li, Y., Zhang, T., Korkaya, H., Liu, S., Lee, H. F., Newman, B., Yu, Y., Clouthier, S. G., Schwartz, S. J., Wicha, M. S., & Sun, D. (2010). Sulforaphane, a Dietary Component of Broccoli/Broccoli Sprouts,

Inhibits Breast Cancer Stem Cells. *Clinical Cancer Research, 16*(9), 2580–2590. https://doi.org/10.1158/1078-0432.ccr-09-2937

Lin, S., Oliveira, M. L., Gabel, K., Kalam, F., Cienfuegos, S., Ezpeleta, M., Bhutani, S., & Varady, K. A. (2020). Does the weight loss efficacy of alternate day fasting differ according to sex and menopausal status? *Nutrition, Metabolism and Cardiovascular Diseases, 31*(2). https://doi.org/10.1016/j.numecd.2020.10.018

Lindberg, S. (2018, August 23). *Autophagy: Definition, diet, fasting, cancer, benefits, and more.* Healthline. https://www.healthline.com/health/autophagy#diet

Lindberg, S. (2020, September 1). *How to exercise safely during intermittent fasting.* Healthline. https://www.healthline.com/health/how-to-exercise-safely-intermittent-fasting

Long, K. (2021, November 18). *Intermittent fasting may protect the heart by controlling inflammation.* American Heart Association. https://www.heart.org/en/news/2021/11/18/intermittent-fasting-may-protect-the-heart-by-controlling-inflammation

Longo, Valter D., & Mattson, Mark P. (2014). Fasting: Molecular Mechanisms and Clinical Applications. *Cell Metabolism, 19*(2), 181–192. https://doi.org/10.1016/j.cmet.2013.12.008

Mahady, G. B., Pendland, S. L., Stoia, A., Hamill, F. A., Fabricant, D., Dietz, B. M., & Chadwick, L. R. (2005). In vitro susceptibility of Helicobacter pylori to botanical extracts used traditionally for the treatment of gastrointestinal disorders. *Phytotherapy Research: PTR, 19*(11), 988–991. https://doi.org/10.1002/ptr.1776

Malinowski, B., Zalewska, K., Węsierska, A., Sokołowska, M. M., Socha, M., Liczner, G., Pawlak-Osińska, K., & Wiciński, M. (2019). Intermittent Fasting in Cardiovascular Disorders-An Overview. *Nutrients, 11*(3), 673. https://doi.org/10.3390/nu11030673

Manoogian, E. N. C., Chaix, A., & Panda, S. (2019). When to Eat: The Importance of Eating Patterns in Health and Disease. *Journal of Biological Rhythms, 34*(6), 579–581. https://doi.org/10.1177/0748730419892105

Manzanero, S., Erion, J. R., Santro, T., Steyn, F. J., Chen, C., Arumugam, T. V., & Stranahan, A. M. (2014). Intermittent Fasting Attenuates Increases in Neurogenesis after Ischemia and Reperfusion and Improves Recovery. *Journal of Cerebral Blood Flow & Metabolism, 34*(5), 897–905. https://doi.org/10.1038/jcbfm.2014.36

Mark Batterson quote (n.d.). Quotefancy. https://quotefancy.com/quote/1528972/Mark-Batterson-You-are-only-one-defining-decision-away-from-a-totally-different-life

Martin, B., Mattson, M. P., & Maudsley, S. (2006). Caloric restriction and intermittent fasting: Two potential diets for successful brain aging. *Ageing Research Reviews, 5*(3), 332–353. https://doi.org/10.1016/j.arr.2006.04.002

Martin, B., Pearson, M., Brenneman, R., Golden, E., Wood, W., Prabhu, V., Becker, K. G., Mattson, M. P., & Maudsley, S. (2009). Gonadal Transcriptome Alterations in Response to Dietary Energy Intake: Sensing the Reproductive Environment. *PLoS ONE, 4*(1), e4146. https://doi.org/10.1371/journal.pone.0004146

Martin, B., Pearson, M., Kebejian, L., Golden, E., Keselman, A., Bender, M., Carlson, O., Egan, J., Ladenheim, B., Cadet, J.-L., Becker, K. G., Wood, W., Duffy, K., Vinayakumar, P., Maudsley, S., & Mattson, M. P. (2007). Sex-Dependent Metabolic, Neuroendocrine, and Cognitive Responses to Dietary Energy Restriction and Excess. *Endocrinology, 148*(9), 4318–4333. https://doi.org/10.1210/en.2007-0161

Martin, S., Hardy, T., & Tollefsbol, T. (2013). Medicinal Chemistry of the Epigenetic Diet and Caloric Restriction. *Current Medicinal*

Chemistry, *20*(32), 4050–4059. https://doi.org/10.2174/09298673113209990189

Mattson, M. P., Longo, V. D., & Harvie, M. (2017). Impact of intermittent fasting on health and disease processes. *Ageing Research Reviews, 39*, 46–58. https://doi.org/10.1016/j.arr.2016.10.005

Mattson, M. P., Moehl, K., Ghena, N., Schmaedick, M., & Cheng, A. (2018). Intermittent metabolic switching, neuroplasticity and brain health. *Nature Reviews Neuroscience, 19*(2), 80–80. https://doi.org/10.1038/nrn.2017.156

Meng, H., Zhu, L., Kord-Varkaneh, H., Santos, H. O., Tinsley, G. M., & Fu, P. (2020). Effects of intermittent fasting and energy-restricted diets on lipid profile: A systematic review and meta-analysis. *Nutrition, 77*, 110801. https://doi.org/10.1016/j.nut.2020.110801

Migala, J. (2020, December 4). *9 amazing health benefits of berries.* Everyday Health. https://www.everydayhealth.com/diet-nutrition-pictures/amazing-health-benefits-of-berries.aspx

Miller, K. (2022, January 6). *8 tips to start intermittent fasting and stick with it.* Women's Health. https://www.womenshealth-mag.com/weight-loss/a38191815/starting-sticking-with-intermittent-fasting/

Mintel Press Team. (2016, May 5). *Super growth for "super" foods: New product development shoots up 202% globally over the past five years.* Mintel. https://www.mintel.com/press-centre/food-and-drink/super-growth-for-super-foods-new-product-development-shoots-up-202-globally-over-the-past-five-years

Morales-Brown, L. (2020, June 11). *Intermittent fasting and exercise: How to do it safely.* Medical News Today. https://www.medicalnewstoday.com/articles/intermittent-fasting-and-working-out

Moro, T., Tinsley, G., Bianco, A., Marcolin, G., Pacelli, Q. F., Battaglia, G., Palma, A., Gentil, P., Neri, M., & Paoli, A. (2016). Effects of eight weeks of time-restricted feeding (16/8) on basal metabolism, maximal strength, body composition, inflammation, and cardiovascular risk factors in resistance-trained males. *Journal of Translational Medicine, 14*(1). https://doi.org/10.1186/s12967-016-1044-0

Mozaffarian, D., Hao, T., Rimm, E. B., Willett, W. C., & Hu, F. B. (2011). Changes in diet and lifestyle and long-term weight gain in women and men. *The New England Journal of Medicine, 364*(25), 2392–2404. https://doi.org/10.1056/NEJMoa1014296

Mudge, L. (2022, May 19). *Intermittent fasting for women: Is it safe?* Live Science. https://www.livescience.com/intermittent-fasting-for-women

Mudryj, A. N., Yu, N., & Aukema, H. M. (2014). Nutritional and health benefits of pulses. *Applied Physiology, Nutrition, and Metabolism, 39*(11), 1197–1204. https://doi.org/10.1139/apnm-2013-0557

Nair, P. M. K., & Khawale, P. G. (2016). Role of therapeutic fasting in women's health: An overview. *Journal of Mid-Life Health, 7*(2), 61. https://doi.org/10.4103/0976-7800.185325

Nazish, N. (2021, June 30). *10 Intermittent fasting myths you should stop believing.* Forbes. https://www.forbes.com/sites/nomanazish/2021/06/30/10-intermittent-fasting-myths-you-should-stop-believing/?sh=420b5a21335b

Netshiomvani, T. (2022, August 13). *14 intermittent fasting benefits, tips, side effects, advice to avoid.* FCER.org. https://fcer.org/intermittent-fasting-benefits/

NIH. (2019). *Calculate your BMI - Metric BMI calculator.* https://www.nhlbi.nih.gov/health/educational/lose_wt/BMI/bmi-m.htm

Ooi, C. P., & Loke, S. C. (2013). Sweet potato for type 2 diabetes mellitus. *Cochrane Database of Systematic Reviews, 9.* https://doi.org/10.1002/14651858.cd009128.pub3

Pannell, N. (2018, August 28). *10 things you've heard about intermittent fasting that aren't true.* Insider. https://www.insider.com/intermittent-fasting-myths-2018-8

Patikorn, C., Roubal, K., Veettil, S. K., Chandran, V., Pham, T., Lee, Y. Y., Giovannucci, E. L., Varady, K. A., & Chaiyakunapruk, N. (2021). Intermittent Fasting and Obesity-Related Health Outcomes. *JAMA Network Open, 4*(12), e2139558. https://doi.org/10.1001/jamanetworkopen.2021.39558

Patterson, R. E., & Sears, D. D. (2017). Metabolic Effects of Intermittent Fasting. *Annual Review of Nutrition, 37*(1), 371–393. https://doi.org/10.1146/annurev-nutr-071816-064634

Patterson, R. E., Laughlin, G. A., LaCroix, A. Z., Hartman, S. J., Natarajan, L., Senger, C. M., Martínez, M. E., Villaseñor, A., Sears, D. D., Marinac, C. R., & Gallo, L. C. (2015). Intermittent Fasting and Human Metabolic Health. *Journal of the Academy of Nutrition and Dietetics, 115*(8), 1203–1212. https://doi.org/10.1016/j.jand.2015.02.018

Petry, N. M., Barry, D., Pietrzak, R. H., & Wagner, J. A. (2008). Overweight and obesity are associated with psychiatric disorders: Results from the national epidemiologic survey on alcohol and related conditions. *Psychosomatic Medicine, 70*(3), 288–297. https://doi.org/10.1097/psy.0b013e3181651651

Prospect Medical. (n.d.). *Working out while intermittent fasting.* https://www.prospectmedical.com/resources/wellness-center/working-out-while-intermittent-fasting

Putka, S. (2021, April 16). *Four ways fasting may help your brain.* Inverse.   https://www.inverse.com/mind-body/how-fasting-affects-the-mind-and-the-body

Ratliff, J., Leite, J. O., de Ogburn, R., Puglisi, M. J., VanHeest, J., & Fernandez, M. L. (2010). Consuming eggs for breakfast influences plasma glucose and ghrelin, while reducing energy intake during the next 24 hours in adult men. *Nutrition Research (New York, N.Y.), 30*(2), 96–103. https://doi.org/10.1016/j.nutres.2010.01.002

Ravichanthiran, K., Ma, Z. F., Zhang, H., Cao, Y., Wang, C. W., Muhammad, S., Aglago, E. K., Zhang, Y., Jin, Y., & Pan, B. (2018). Phytochemical Profile of Brown Rice and Its Nutrigenomic Implications.   *Antioxidants,*   7(6),   71. https://doi.org/10.3390/antiox7060071

Remedies for keto flu. (2020, December 2). WebMD. https://www.webmd.com/diet/remedies-for-keto-flu#1

Richard, C., Cristall, L., Fleming, E., Lewis, E. D., Ricupero, M., Jacobs, R. L., & Field, C. J. (2017). Impact of Egg Consumption on Cardiovascular Risk Factors in Individuals with Type 2 Diabetes and at Risk for Developing Diabetes: A Systematic Review of Randomized Nutritional Intervention Studies. *Canadian Journal of Diabetes, 41*(4), 453–463. https://doi.org/10.1016/j.jcjd.2016.12.002

Ries, J. (2020, March 24). *What are probiotics actually good for? We asked the experts.* Greatist. https://greatist.com/health/should-i-take-a-probiotic

Rizzo, N. (2022, January 30). *What foods are best to eat on an intermittent fasting diet?* Greatist. https://greatist.com/eat/what-to-eat-on-an-intermittent-fasting-diet#foods-to-eat-on-if

Robertson, R. (2020, October 22). *Omega-3-6-9 fatty acids: A complete overview*. Healthline. https://www.healthline.com/nutrition/omega-3-6-9-overview#omega-6

Rosa, D. D., Dias, M. M. S., Grześkowiak, Ł. M., Reis, S. A., Conceição, L. L., & Peluzio, M. do C. G. (2017). Milk kefir: nutritional, microbiological and health benefits. *Nutrition Research Reviews, 30*(1), 82–96. https://doi.org/10.1017/s0954422416000275

Rowles, A. (2017, June 7). *Why liver is a nutrient-dense superfood*. Healthline. https://www.healthline.com/nutrition/why-liver-is-a-superfood

Sadiya, A., Ahmed, Siddieg, Joy, & Carlsson. (2011). Effect of Ramadan fasting on metabolic markers, body composition, and dietary intake in Emiratis of Ajman (UAE) with metabolic syndrome. *Diabetes, Metabolic Syndrome and Obesity: Targets and Therapy*, 409. https://doi.org/10.2147/dmso.s24221

Sales-Campos, H., Souza, P. R. de, Peghini, B. C., da Silva, J. S., & Cardoso, C. R. (2013). An overview of the modulatory effects of oleic acid in health and disease. *Mini Reviews in Medicinal Chemistry, 13*(2), 201–210. https://pubmed.ncbi.nlm.nih.gov/23278117/

Santos, H. O., & Macedo, R. C. O. (2018). Impact of intermittent fasting on the lipid profile: Assessment associated with diet and weight loss. *Clinical Nutrition ESPEN, 24*, 14–21. https://doi.org/10.1016/j.clnesp.2018.01.002

Schwartz, M. (2020, September 24). *3 benefits of fasting for a healthy gut*. Health. https://www.health.com/nutrition/how-to-fast-healthy-gut

Seimon, R. V., Roekenes, J. A., Zibellini, J., Zhu, B., Gibson, A. A., Hills, A. P., Wood, R. E., King, N. A., Byrne, N. M., & Sainsbury, A. (2015). Do intermittent diets provide physiological benefits over continuous diets for weight loss? A systematic review of clinical trials. *Molecular and Cellular Endocrinology, 418*, 153–172. https://doi.org/10.1016/j.mce.2015.09.014

7 incredible things intermittent fasting does for your brain. (2020, March 2). Amen Clinics. https://www.amenclinics.com/blog/7-incredible-things-intermittent-fasting-does-for-your-brain/

Shi, H., Zhang, B., Abo-Hamzy, T., Nelson, J. W., Ambati, C. S. R., Petrosino, J. F., Bryan, Jr., R. M., & Durgan, D. J. (2021). Restructuring the Gut Microbiota by Intermittent Fasting Lowers Blood Pressure. *Circulation Research, 128*(9). https://doi.org/10.1161/circresaha.120.318155

Shojaie, M., Ghanbari, F., & Shojaie, N. (2017). Intermittent fasting could ameliorate cognitive function against distress by regulation of inflammatory response pathway. *Journal of Advanced Research, 8*(6), 697–701. https://doi.org/10.1016/j.jare.2017.09.002

Simon, G. E., Von Korff, M., Saunders, K., Miglioretti, D. L., Crane, P. K., van Belle, G., & Kessler, R. C. (2006). Association Between Obesity and Psychiatric Disorders in the US Adult Population. *Archives of General Psychiatry, 63*(7), 824. https://doi.org/10.1001/archpsyc.63.7.824

Sköldstam, L., Larsson, L., & Lindström, F. D. (1979). Effect of fasting and lactovegetarian diet on rheumatoid arthritis. *Scandinavian Journal of Rheumatology, 8*(4), 249–255. https://doi.org/10.3109/03009747909114631

Skrovankova, S., Sumczynski, D., Mlcek, J., Jurikova, T., & Sochor, J. (2015). Bioactive Compounds and Antioxidant Activity in Different Types of Berries. *International Journal of Molecular Sciences, 16*(10), 24673–24706. https://doi.org/10.3390/ijms161024673

Snyder, C. (2022, February 23). *5 intermittent fasting methods, reviewed.* Healthline. https://www.healthline.com/nutrition/6-ways-to-do-intermittent-fasting?utm_source=ReadNext#bottom-line

Sodium in diet: MedlinePlus Medical Encyclopedia. (n.d.). MedlinePlus. https://medlineplus.gov/ency/article/002415.htm

Soeters, M. R., Sauerwein, H. P., Groener, J. E., Aerts, J. M., Ackermans, M. T., Glatz, J. F. C., Fliers, E., & Serlie, M. J. (2007). Gender-related differences in the metabolic response to fasting. *The Journal of Clinical Endocrinology and Metabolism, 92*(9), 3646–3652. https://doi.org/10.1210/jc.2007-0552

Solianik, R., & Sujeta, A. (2018). Two-day fasting evokes stress, but does not affect mood, brain activity, cognitive, psychomotor, and motor performance in overweight women. *Behavioural Brain Research, 338,* 166–172. https://doi.org/10.1016/j.bbr.2017.10.028

Solianik, R., Sujeta, A., Terentjevienė, A., & Skurvydas, A. (2016). Effect of 48 h Fasting on Autonomic Function, Brain Activity, Cognition, and Mood in Amateur Weight Lifters. *BioMed Research International, 2016,* 1–8. https://doi.org/10.1155/2016/1503956

Stekovic, S., Hofer, S. J., Tripolt, N., Aon, M. A., Royer, P., Pein, L., Stadler, J. T., Pendl, T., Prietl, B., Url, J., Schroeder, S., Tadic, J., Eisenberg, T., Magnes, C., Stumpe, M., Zuegner, E., Bordag, N., Riedl, R., Schmidt, A., & Kolesnik, E. (2019). Alternate Day Fasting Improves Physiological and Molecular Markers of Aging in Healthy, Non-obese Humans. *Cell Metabolism, 30*(3), 462-476.e5. https://doi.org/10.1016/j.cmet.2019.07.016

Stevenson, J. L., Paton, C. M., & Cooper, J. A. (2017). Hunger and satiety responses to high-fat meals after a high-polyunsaturated fat diet: A randomized trial. *Nutrition, 41,* 14–23. https://doi.org/10.1016/j.nut.2017.03.008

Stockman, M.-C., Thomas, D., Burke, J., & Apovian, C. M. (2018). Intermittent Fasting: Is the Wait Worth the Weight? Current Obesity Reports, 7(2), 172–185. https://doi.org/10.1007/s13679-018-0308-9

Stone, J. (2018, November 22). *What is ketogenesis? Are ketosis and ketogenesis the same?* Shortcut to Ketosis. https://shortcutketo.com/ketogenesis-in-low-glucose-levels/

Stote, K. S., Baer, D. J., Spears, K., Paul, D. R., Harris, G. K., Rumpler, W. V., Strycula, P., Najjar, S. S., Ferrucci, L., Ingram, D. K., Longo, D. L., & Mattson, M. P. (2007). A controlled trial of reduced meal frequency without caloric restriction in healthy, normal-weight, middle-aged adults. *The American Journal of Clinical Nutrition,* *85*(4), 981–988. https://doi.org/10.1093/ajcn/85.4.981

Sundfør, T. M., Svendsen, M., & Tonstad, S. (2018). Effect of intermittent versus continuous energy restriction on weight loss, maintenance and cardiometabolic risk: A randomized 1-year trial. *Nutrition, Metabolism and Cardiovascular Diseases,* 28(7), 698–706. https://doi.org/10.1016/j.numecd.2018.03.009

Sutton, E. F., Beyl, R., Early, K. S., Cefalu, W. T., Ravussin, E., & Peterson, C. M. (2018). Early Time-Restricted Feeding Improves Insulin Sensitivity, Blood Pressure, and Oxidative Stress Even without Weight Loss in Men with Prediabetes. *Cell Metabolism,* *27*(6), 1212-1221.e3. https://doi.org/10.1016/j.cmet.2018.04.010

Tanaka, T., Shnimizu, M., & Moriwaki, H. (2012). Cancer chemoprevention by carotenoids. *Molecules (Basel, Switzerland),* *17*(3), 3202–3242. https://doi.org/10.3390/molecules17033202

Templeman, I., Thompson, D., Gonzalez, J., Walhin, J.-P., Reeves, S., Rogers, P. J., Brunstrom, J. M., Karagounis, L. G., Tsintzas, K., & Betts, J. A. (2018). Intermittent fasting, energy balance and associated health outcomes in adults: study protocol for a randomised controlled trial. *Trials, 19*(1), 86. https://doi.org/10.1186/s13063-018-2451-8

The 10 best intermittent fasting tips and tricks. (2018, October 31). Lift Learn Grow. https://www.liftlearngrow.com/blog-page/best-intermittent-fasting-tips/

The effects of intermittent fasting on brain function. (2017, August 8). Shine+. https://shinedrink.com/blogs/brainbites/the-effects-of-intermittent-fasting-on-brain-function#:~:text=All%20indications%20show%20that%20intermittent

32 top intermittent fasting recipes. (n.d.). Food.com https://www.-food.com/ideas/intermittent-fasting-recipes-6939#c-798501

Tinsley, G. M., Forsse, J. S., Butler, N. K., Paoli, A., Bane, A. A., La Bounty, P. M., Morgan, G. B., & Grandjean, P. W. (2016). Time-restricted feeding in young men performing resistance training: A randomized controlled trial. *European Journal of Sport Science, 17*(2), 200–207. https://doi.org/10.1080/17461391.2016.1223173

Trumpfeller, G. (2020, July 22). *Do you need to take supplements during intermittent fasting?* Simple. https://simple.life/blog/intermittent-fasting-and-supplements/

Try our recipe nutrition calculator. (n.d.). Verywell Fit. https://www.verywellfit.com/recipe-nutrition-analyzer-4157076

USDA. (2019, April 1). *FoodData Central.* https://fdc.-nal.usda.gov/fdc-app.html#/food-details/174250/nutrients

USDA. (2020). *Dietary guidelines for Americans 2020–2025.* https://www.dietaryguidelines.gov/sites/default/files/2021-03/Dietary_Guidelines_for_Americans-2020-2025.pdf

Varady, K. A. (2011). Intermittent versus daily calorie restriction: which diet regimen is more effective for weight loss? *Obesity*

178   *References*

Reviews, 12(7), e593–e601. https://doi.org/10.1111/j.1467-789x.2011.00873.x

Varady, K. A., Bhutani, S., Church, E. C., & Klempel, M. C. (2009). Short-term modified alternate-day fasting: a novel dietary strategy for weight loss and cardioprotection in obese adults. *The American Journal of Clinical Nutrition, 90*(5), 1138–1143. https://doi.org/10.3945/ajcn.2009.28380

Varady, K. A., Bhutani, S., Klempel, M. C., Kroeger, C. M., Trepanowski, J. F., Haus, J. M., Hoddy, K. K., & Calvo, Y. (2013). Alternate day fasting for weight loss in normal weight and overweight subjects: a randomized controlled trial. *Nutrition Journal, 12*(1). https://doi.org/10.1186/1475-2891-12-146

Varady, K. A., Cienfuegos, S., Ezpeleta, M., & Gabel, K. (2021). Cardiometabolic Benefits of Intermittent Fasting. *Annual Review of Nutrition, 41*(1), 333–361. https://doi.org/10.1146/annurev-nutr-052020-041327

Veronese, N., & Reginster, J.-Y. (2019). The effects of calorie restriction, intermittent fasting and vegetarian diets on bone health. *Aging Clinical and Experimental Research, 31*(6), 753–758. https://doi.org/10.1007/s40520-019-01174-x

Vetter, C. (2022, January 26). *Intermittent fasting for women: Here's what you need to know.* ZOE. https://joinzoe.com/learn/intermittent-fasting-for-women

Vieira, A. F., Costa, R. R., Macedo, R. C. O., Coconcelli, L., & Kruel, L. F. M. (2016). Effects of aerobic exercise performed in fasted v. fed state on fat and carbohydrate metabolism in adults: a systematic review and meta-analysis. *British Journal of Nutrition, 116*(7), 1153–1164. https://doi.org/10.1017/s0007114516003160

Wang, C., Harris, W. S., Chung, M., Lichtenstein, A. H., Balk, E. M., Kupelnick, B., Jordan, H. S., & Lau, J. (2006). n−3 Fatty acids from